Risk-takers

KT-365-948

Adolescence is a turbulent period, a time when young people are particularly prone to risky behaviours, such as drug use and unprotected sex. *Risk-takers* provides a comprehensive view of youthful involvement with drinking, smoking, illicit drug use and sexual activity. In particular, the authors explore the evidence linking alcohol, drug use, 'disinhibition' and risky sex.

They discuss these issues in relation to evidence suggesting that some forms of risk-taking are interconnected. Though some young people are especially prone to take risks due to poverty and social disadvantage, the authors emphasize that risk-taking is commonplace adolescent behaviour, difficult to restrain or curb. They remind us that past attempts to reduce youthful alcohol and drug misuse have produced disappointing results, and they also point out that most young people have not modified their sexual behaviour in the light of the risks of AIDS.

Risk-taking is unlikely to be prevented by mass media campaigns or bland slogans such as 'Just Say No'. The authors examine the effectiveness of preventive strategies and public policy and emphasize the importance of 'harm minimization' strategies. This review provides a challenging assessment of health-threatening behaviours among young people.

Risk-takers
Alcohol, drugs, sex and youth

Martin Plant and Moira Plant

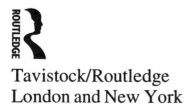

Tavistock/Routledge
London and New York

First published in 1992
by Routledge
11 New Fetter Lane, London EC4P 4EE

Simultaneously published in the USA and Canada
by Routledge
a division of Routledge, Chapman and Hall, Inc.
29 West 35th Street, New York, NY 10001

© 1992 Martin Plant and Moira Plant

Typeset in Times by LaserScript Limited, Mitcham, Surrey
Printed and bound in Great Britain by
Biddles Ltd, Guildford and King's Lynn

All rights reserved. No part of this book may be reprinted
or reproduced or utilized in any form or by any electronic, mechanical,
or other means, now known or hereafter invented, including
photocopying and recording, or in any information storage
or retrieval system, without permission in writing from the publishers.

British Library Cataloguing in Publication Data
A catalogue record for this book is available from the British Library.

Library of Congress Cataloging in Publication Data
Plant, Martin A.
    Risk-takers : alcohol, drugs, sex and youth / Martin Plant and Moira Plant.
    p.   cm.
Includes bibliographical references and index.
1. Teenagers – Great Britain.   2. Risk-taking (Psychology) in adolescence –
Great Britain.   3. Teenagers – Great Britain – Sexual behaviour.   4. Teenagers –
Great Britain – Alcohol use.   5. Teenagers – Great Britain – Drug use.   I. Plant,
Moira. II. Title.
HQ799.G7P54 1992
305.23'5'0941–dc20   91–41467
                                                                          CIP

ISBN 0–415–03538–4 (hbk)
        0–415–03539–2 (pbk)

This book is dedicated to Emma Judith Plant

Contents

Figures and tables

The authors

Martin Plant PhD is Director of the Alcohol Research Group in the University of Edinburgh. Dr Plant, a sociologist, has been engaged in research into the use and misuse of legal and illegal drugs since 1970. His publications include *Drugtakers in an English Town*; *Drinking Careers*; *Alcohol, Drugs and School-leavers* and *Drugs in Perspective*. He has edited several books, including *Economics and Alcohol*; *Drinking and Problem Drinking*; *AIDS, Drugs and Prostitution*; *Alcohol and Drugs: Research and Policy* and *Alcohol and Drugs: The Scottish Experience*. He was a co-author of the Royal College of Psychiatrists' reports *Alcohol: Our Favourite Drug* and *Drug Scenes*.

Moira Plant PhD is a Research Fellow in the Alcohol Research Group in the University of Edinburgh. She is a psychiatric nurse and psychotherapist and was Charge Nurse in the Alcohol Problems Clinic (formerly the Unit for the Treatment of Alcoholism) in the Royal Edinburgh Hospital between 1971 and 1978. She has been a member of the Alcohol Research Group since 1980. Her publications include the book *Women, Drinking and Pregnancy* and the report *Women and Alcohol*. Her recent research relates to alcohol, stress and nursing and to AIDS risks in the sex industry. Moira Plant is a member of the Government working group on Women and Alcohol.

Acknowledgements

The authors are greatly indebted to many people and agencies for assistance with the compilation of the material presented in this book. Particular thanks are due to the following for the provision of information, some of it hitherto unpublished, and for permission to cite: Dr Phillip Aitken, Mr Niall Coggans, Professor John B. Davies, Dr Julian Everest, Dr Nicholas Ford, Dr Pamela Gillies, Ms. Eileen Goddard, Dr Richard Jessor, Dr Barbara Leigh, Mr Robert McEwan, Dr Alexander McMillan, Mr David Mason, Dr Carl May, Mr Roger Penwill, Mr Craig Smith, Professor Gerry Stimson, Mr Chris Thurman, Mr Peter Weatherburn, Mr Noel Williams, Action on Smoking and Health, the Brewers' Society, the Department of Health, the Department of Social Security, the Department of Transport, the *Dundee Courier and Advertiser*, the Health Education Authority, the Health Education Board for Scotland, the Institute for the Study of Drug Dependence, LRC Products Ltd, Lothian Health Board, the Office of Population Censuses and Surveys and the World Health Organization. Figures 12.1 and 12.2 are crown copyright. These are reproduced with permission from the Controller of Her Majesty's Stationery Office.

Thanks go to Mrs Joyce Greig, Mrs Sheila McLennan and Mrs Janis Nichol for their amiable and efficient word processing from an illegible text.

Introduction

This book, as the title suggests, sets out to provide an overview of two major areas of 'risky behaviour' in relation to young people. The first of these relates to the use and misuse of legal and illicit drugs. The second relates to sexual behaviour. It is emphasized that, while risk-taking amongst adolescents is quite normal, most young people do not expose themselves to major risks. The great majority of those who drink do so in moderation. Most young people in Britain, and in several other countries, do not smoke tobacco or use illicit drugs. In addition, growing awareness of the spreading AIDS epidemic has certainly exerted an influence, though often only a marginal one, on the sexual behaviour of adolescents and young adults. This book sets out to put 'risk-taking' into a balanced perspective. This necessitates the presentation of a general account of recent evidence related to both the use and the misuse of alcohol, tobacco and illicit drugs and of research evidence related to sexual behaviour and to various forms of risk-taking.

There are so many books about alcohol, tobacco and drugs, why write yet another? Perhaps the best reply to this question is to acknowledge that fashions in drinking, smoking and other forms of mind-altering substance use continually change. Accordingly, each thesis, report or book on this subject tends to have a relatively short shelf-life and to become a historical, rather than a current, contribution in a matter of weeks or months. Books about sexual behaviour and the AIDS epidemic probably become outdated even more quickly than books about drinking habits or other forms of drug use.

The main focus of this book is 'young people'. For the purposes of this text 'young people' are taken to be those aged 21 or below. In fact it is freely admitted that the information presented below includes numerous departures from this definition. When the authors judge it to be appropriate reference is also made to people above the age of 21.

A variety of terms has been applied to encompass 'young people'. These include 'children', 'teenagers' and 'adolescents'. These terms may all be defined in relation to age or to other factors. A useful reminder of the social and cultural variation implicit in such definitions, as well as the complexities of such concepts, has been provided by Baumrind:

Our culture has no rites of passage to demarcate the change in status from child to adult, but it has instead a long transitional period that we call adolescence. By adolescence I refer to an age span roughly between ages ten and twenty-five that is heralded by the accelerating physical changes accompanying puberty; results in sexual maturity and identity formation; and eventuates in emancipation from childhood dependency and crucial decisions concerning school, love and work. Adolescence is a psychosocial stage in the lifespan and therefore specific to class and culture.

(Baumrind 1987: 97)

Human beings have a widespread and long-standing affinity for alcohol, tobacco, cannabis, opiates and allied substances. Most people are in some way drug users and the value of such substances is underlined by the voracious demand for them. Sadly, humans are not always rational or careful in their ways. Drug taking is all too often complicated by inappropriate or harmful use. It is doubtful if there is any such entity as a 'safe drug'. Even the most familiar and innocuous substance appears to be used in a harmful manner by some people, even if these constitute only a small minority of users. 'Drug misuse', 'drug problems' or 'drug abuse' appear to be the inevitable price that is incurred by humanity's liking for chemical methods of mood adaptation. At its most extreme such misuse is illustrated by the plight and dereliction of Skid Row meths drinkers, the misery of housewives unable to face another day without yet another prescription for tranquillizers, the middle-aged smoker dying from lung cancer and emphysema or of the young man or woman dying of AIDS contracted by the sharing of infected injecting equipment or by unprotected sexual contact.

Equally tragic is the toll of injury and death inflicted by alcohol-related accidents and violence. In fact, drug use does not occur in isolation and the precise role of drugs, legal or illegal, in specific health or social problems is often unclear. For example, it has been alleged that young soccer fans fight because they have been drinking: plenty of people drink without fighting and alcohol consumption is not in itself an adequate explanation for violence, even if it is frequently an associated or possible contributory factor.

Sexual behaviour is also one of the main themes of this book and in particular the connection between 'risky' sex and the use of alcohol and drugs such as cannabis, amphetamines and cocaine. Legal and illegal drug use have long been linked with sexuality for a host of reasons. These include social and cultural as well as psychological and physiological factors. Drinking is commonly associated with dating and with sexual encounters. So too are a number of 'illicit drugs', albeit on a less popular or widespread basis.

During recent years the connection between 'risky sex' and psychoactive drugs has been accorded vastly added seriousness by the advent of the AIDS epidemic. This is not the first time that humanity has been confronted by the spectre of a sexually transmitted disease which is incurable and fatal. Even so, while the search for a 'cure' for AIDS continues, particular attention is, quite logically, being paid to determining which factors foster the spread of HIV infection and to possible ways of curbing such spread. Since the upsurge of HIV infection in industrial countries it has been obvious that intravenous drug use, in particular the sharing of infected injecting equipment, is a major risk factor. More recently, attention has been drawn to the possible role of alcohol and other 'disinhibiting' substances in relation to high risk or unprotected sex.

The review that is presented of alcohol, tobacco and illicit drug use and related problems is written from a largely British perspective. Even so, it is hoped that when appropriate more general information is also cited, especially in the consideration of the crucial, practical topics of 'prevention' and 'harm minimization'. The chapters related to sexual behaviour, drugs and pregnancy, alcohol, drugs and risky sex and risk-taking draw heavily upon evidence not only from Britain but also from the USA and elsewhere.

1 The causes of drug use

This book is primarily concerned with the youthful use and misuse of alcohol, tobacco and illicit drugs and with the sexual behaviour of young people. As a preliminary to the presentation of a selective review of some of the evidence related to these topics it is considered important to provide readers with a brief introduction to the many possible reasons why people sometimes use and misuse psychoactive (mind-altering) drugs. Such drugs, it should be noted, include alcohol, tobacco and prescribed as well as illicit drugs.

The inclusion of this chapter may seem anomalous. It is the authors' intention to include it for two reasons. Firstly, the complexity of the factors that influence human risk-taking is crucial to any understanding of such behaviour. Secondly, the aetiology, not only of drug use, but of other potentially harmful behaviours has to be taken into account when considering realistic ways of minimizing risk-taking by young people.

'Drugs' are frequently portrayed by the mass media as inherently harmful, injurious and malign. This impression, reasonably enough, is clearly reinforced by stereotypes of the casualties of various form of damaging drug use. Such stereotypes, the 'wino', the 'alcoholic' and 'the junkie', are frequently held up as cautionary representations, and combined with warnings about the perils of excess or deviant forms of drug use. Simple images often beget simple solutions. Messages such as 'Just Say No!' have both clarity and a popular appeal. In fact, neither drug use nor other health-related behaviours conform to convenient stereotypes. Moreover, there are, as yet, no simple magic solutions whereby harmful behaviours may be prevented. Human behaviour is as varied and confusing as its attendant problems and negative consequences abound.

The following chapters present, from the authors' perspective, an overview of some of the recent evidence related to psychoactive drug use and sexual behaviour in relation to young people. Alcohol and drug use and sexual behaviour are influenced by many factors. The existence of these factors has profound implications for policies intended to reduce, even to prevent, harmful drug use or the adverse consequences of unprotected sex.

This chapter does not provide a detailed and comprehensive review of evidence and theories related to the aetiology of drug use and drug dependence. More complete reviews are available elsewhere (e.g. Fazey 1977; Plant 1981; Peck 1982). Theories abound. They may be broadly divided into constitutional or biological, individual and environmental.

CONSTITUTIONAL FACTORS

Constitutional or biological theories are related to biological predispositions to use or to misuse drugs or with the physical effects of their use. For example, animal research has indicated the existence of genetic predispositions to use drugs or to become dependent upon them. There is also some evidence in humans indicating that some people are predisposed to develop such problems as liver disease, alcohol dependence or certain types of cancers. It has been suggested that specific individuals, due to biological or psychological traits, are particularly attracted to stimulant, depressant or hallucinogenic drugs. Some people like particular drug effects. Such theories need to be considered in relation to a host of other individual factors, as well as social and cultural factors. If alcohol problems run in families, this could be for social as well as biological reasons (Goodwin 1976; Partanen, Bruun and Markkanen 1966; Kiianmaa, Tabakoff and Saito 1989; Kozlowski 1991).

INDIVIDUAL FACTORS

Personality

A considerable amount of work has been conducted to identify an 'addictive personality'. The resulting evidence is contradictory. Many of these results stem from studies which have compared those who use alcohol or illicit drugs in a problematic way with 'control groups' of different types. Often the latter have been chosen from rather unusual groups of people. These include those in penal institutions and clinic patients. Some studies have suggested that problem drinkers or problem drug users do differ from controls in relation to psychological characteristics such as neuroticism, hostility or extraversion. Even so, no unique 'alcohol-dependent' or 'drug-dependent' personality has been delineated (Fazey 1977; Plant 1981).

Gender

In most societies males use drugs more than do females. Even so, as elaborated in Chapters 2–7, there are exceptions to this rule. Females are as likely or, in some cases, more likely than males to use or to misuse specific drugs. For example, males in Britain drink more than females, but the latter are more likely than males to take prescribed tranquillizers. Social mores which once constrained women from drinking and using other drugs have been changing. This has been reflected by a change in the genders' relative positions with regard to patterns of drug use. This is elaborated in Chapters 2–7.

Age

This book is concerned with 'young people'. It is clear that the young are more likely than older people to use illicit drugs. The young, however, are less likely than their forebears to smoke. As emphasized constantly throughout this book, the young are, by virtue of their relative inexperience, possibly more likely to get into difficulties than older people in relation to psychoactive drug use. In addition, adolescents may well be more inclined than older people to take risks, to test out their limits to the full. Sometimes such risk-taking involves serious drug misuse (Jessor and Jessor 1977; Stimson 1981; MacGregor 1989).

Intelligence

Most drug misusers are not stupid. Some are from severely disadvantaged backgrounds, others are not. Various studies support the conclusion that neither the use nor the misuse of legal or illicit drugs can be attributed to low intelligence or to lack of information.

Psychological health

Some of those with serious alcohol or other drug problems have serious psychological disorders. It is often extremely difficult to tell whether these disorders are a cause or a result of the alcohol or drug use. Sometimes an alcohol or a drug problem appears to be at least partly caused by a secondary psychological condition. Studies of institutionalized problem drinkers and problem drug users vary considerably in their findings, with differing levels of association between psychoactive drug problems and psychological ill health (e.g. Kraft 1970; Barnes and Noble 1972; Lane 1976; Silver 1977).

Stressful life events

Clinical studies have commonly noted a high level of stressful life events amongst those with serious alcohol and drug problems. Such connections may reflect the fact that stressful life events may be caused by or result from alcohol and drug misuse. In addition, it is possible that difficult life circumstances may combine to produce both such life events and heavy or problematic psychoactive drug use (e.g. Ogborne 1975; Melotte 1975; Blumberg 1981).

Risk-taking

'Risk' is one of the major themes of this book. It is emphasized that for many people drinking, smoking, illicit drug use or sexual behaviour are neither perceived as being risky nor do they lead to adverse consequences. Risk-taking is the subject of Chapter 11 and is discussed at length therein. There is evidence to suggest, firstly, that risk-taking is normal amongst young people and, secondly, that some individuals do take more risks than others. In relation to certain behaviours, adolescence appears to be a time of heightened risk-taking (Baumrind 1987).

Hedonism

Most people who use drugs do so because the effects are enjoyable or rewarding in some way. These 'rewards' could be attributable to the chemical/psychological effects of particular drugs or, equally, to their perceived social significance and prestige. Most drug use is recreational or, to at least some extent, motivated by enjoyment.

Self-medication

Clinical studies of those who use drugs heavily or for long periods of time suggest that some drug use is motivated by a wish for self-medication. Many drug users and problem drinkers attribute their behaviours to a wish to attain specific psychological states. These range from euphoria to oblivion. It is not uncommon for heavy drug users to seek drug supplies both legally from medical practitioners and illegally through black market transactions.

Curiosity

Initial drug use has been widely attributed to curiosity (Goode 1970; Davies and Stacey 1972). This is elaborated in Chapters 2, 3 and 4 and applies as much to initial alcohol and tobacco use as it does to the use of illicit drugs. Curiosity is not solely a youthful characteristic, nor does it explain why some people, after drug initiation, continue use or become heavy or problem users. It is emphasized that, while some individuals may be inherently more inquisitive, curious or venturesome than others, curiosity may be strongly influenced by social and cultural factors including, for example, peer pressure and mass media coverage of drug issues.

ENVIRONMENTAL FACTORS

Many theories have been propounded which attempt to relate drug use or misuse to the wider context in which such behaviours take place. A huge body of literature has examined social and cultural factors such as socio-economic status, poverty, truancy, delinquency and family backgrounds. Some studies have sought to identify factors which are linked with drug use in the general population. Others have attempted to distinguish factors associated with atypical or harmful forms of drug use. As noted above, there is a considerable body of evidence that institutionalized problem drinkers and other problem drug users do exhibit high rates of other 'problem' characteristics. The inter-correlation of such problems or types of risky behaviour is central to the material presented in this book and is considered further in Chapter 11.

Socio-economic status/poverty

Patterns of drug use and misuse often vary in relation to socio-economic status. Different sub-groups in society have characteristic fashions in behaviour and this includes the use of legal or illicit drugs. In spite of this, both drug use and drug problems occur at all socio-economic levels. They are *not* the prerogative of the socially disadvantaged or those in extreme poverty. Even so, some forms of drug use and misuse are associated with social deprivation. Areas such as Moss Side in Manchester, the Wirral in Cheshire or Muirhouse in Edinburgh, for example, appear far more likely to foster youthful intravenous drug use than do more affluent areas. Set against this, plenty of affluent people in high status occupations also misuse legal and illicit drugs (Stimson 1981; Royal College of Psychiatrists 1986; MacGregor 1989).

Peer pressure

Studies of the use of drugs by young people repeatedly emphasize the importance of peer pressure in encouraging and maintaining drug use.

Younger children, though usually much influenced by parents and other relatives, are also often subject to peer group influences. The latter become stronger with age and, by the teenage years, typically peer pressure from friends overtakes family influence in relation to styles of alcohol, cigarette and illicit drug use. Societies have 'establishment' or 'conventional' orientations towards issues such as drugs and sex. Typically these promote abstinence or moderation. Youthful peer group pressures may condone and foster very different fashions (Davies and Stacey 1972; Plant 1975; Bagnall 1991c).

Ideology/religion

As a corollary of the previous paragraph drug use may be associated with or proscribed by specific ideologies, creeds or religions. During the 1960s and 1970s illicit drug use was linked in many countries with a spirit of youthful rebellion and with subterranean or counter-cultural values exemplified by the hippy life-style. Much has been written about drugs during this period. It is ironic, but perhaps understandable, that the romanticism of the drug scene at this time coincided with the height of the Cold War and the conflict in Vietnam. Illicit drug use, though compatible with youth protest, was and is incompatible with more conventional beliefs such as those of most of the traditional, orthodox world religions (Young 1971). Some commentators have suggested that adherence to such religions serves to reduce the likelihood of illicit drug use. The role of religion in discouraging alcohol use is clearly demonstrated, not only in Islamic societies, but in the 'Bible Belt' of the USA and in Ireland (Pittman and Snyder 1962).

Troubled families

It has been noted above that stressful life events have been linked with alcohol and drug problems. Considerable evidence also connects such problems with familial disturbance, such as separation from one or both parents, 'broken homes' and parental drug abuse. There is also evidence indicating that if parents are strict non-drinkers this, like parental heavy drinking, fails to provide a model of moderate alcohol use for children to follow. Many clinical studies have noted that those with alcohol and drug problems do report backgrounds of severe family disturbance. Such backgrounds are, it should be noted, not unique to those with substance-related problems. Moreover, it is certainly not the case that all of those with alcohol or drug problems come from unduly troubled or dysfunctional families (e.g. Woodside 1973; Judson 1973; Blumberg 1981; Orford and Harwin 1982).

Education disturbance

Young people who drink, smoke or use illicit drugs are generally un-
remarkable, simply because use of these substances is common. There is,
however, evidence from the USA, Britain and elsewhere that individuals
whose drug use is heavy or problematic frequently have educational problems. These include truancy and early departure from full-time education
(Jessor and Jessor 1977). The topic of truancy is discussed further in
Chapter 11.

Crime

There is abundant evidence that heavy drinking and illicit drug use are
associated with crimes, including violent crimes (e.g. Collins 1982; Myers
1982; Brain 1986). In spite of much extensive research no clear causal
relationship has yet been demonstrated. An *association* may imply many
things. The frequently noted link between alcohol, other drug use and crime
certainly involves the disinhibiting effects of such drugs, which are discussed further in Chapter 10. In addition, this association also involves
other factors such as the characteristics of criminals, heavy drinkers and
drug users and situational or environmental factors. No psychoactive drug
is able to generate criminal behaviours when consumed by individuals who
are not otherwise likely to engage in such acts.

Availability/price

There is no doubt that the price and availability of both legal and illicit
drugs are important influences on patterns of use and misuse. A major
determinant of alcohol and tobacco consumption is the price of these
products in relation to disposable incomes. Fluctuations in legal and illicit
drug consumption reflect a variety of factors. These include attitudes to the
drugs in question and social support for such drug use. Clearly, availability
reflects consumer preferences. Even so, consumer preferences and consumption levels are, in turn, also influenced by price and availability (Plant,
Grant and Williams 1981; Sales *et al.* 1989).

The list of theories put forward to explain legal and illicit drug use and
misuse is almost endless. They include historical, economic, political and
sociological theories. Most, if not all, of these theories are consistent with
at least some examples of drug use. Nevertheless, the complexities and
variety of drug-taking behaviour cannot be adequately explained by any
single theory. It has, for example, even been suggested that there is a basic
human need to experience altered states of consciousness. This may be so,

but such states need not be attained through drug use. Music or meditation, for example, may produce much the same effects. This chapter has not presented either a full or a detailed review of aetiological theories. Table 1.1 indicates only some of the factors which have been suggested as influencing drug use and misuse.

Table 1.1 indicates a number of the factors which have been linked with various forms of psychoactive drug use. Some of these factors, such as curiosity, availability and peer pressure, have frequently been cited as fostering initial drug use or experimentation. Other factors, such as (again) peer pressure together with price and availability, have been linked to continued drug use. 'Abnormal', 'heavy' or problematic drug use has been attributed to a wide range of difficulties or characteristics which imply social and psychological disadvantage. These include stressful life events such as parental separation or divorce, psychological ill health and unemployment.

To conclude, the aetiology of alcohol, tobacco, prescribed and illicit drug use is complex. Fazey (1977) has provided a detailed review of this extremely daunting evidence. The causes of drug use and other risky behaviours have enormous relevance to any consideration of these behaviours and in particular to policies to curb or prevent associated problems. As indicated by the following twelve chapters, potentially risky

Table 1.1 Factors associated with drug use and misuse

Individual factors	Environmental factors	Constituent factors
Personality	Socio-economic status	Biological/genetic
Gender	Poverty	predisposition to
Anxiety	Delinquency	use/misuse drugs
Stress	Family background/	
Power needs	disturbance	
Age	Peer pressure	
Intelligence	Ideology/religion	
Psychological health	Educational opportunities	
Life events	Educational disturbance	
Predisposition to take	Truancy	
risks	Drug availability	
Hedonism	Drug price	
Self-destructiveness	Unemployment/	
Curiosity	job opportunities	
	Anomie	
	Alienation	
	Tradition	
	Legal arrangements	
	Historical factors	

activities are extremely popular amongst young adults. Some, such as the use of illicit drugs and sex, are possibly more popular and widespread than ever before. Most drug use and, certainly, sexual behaviours are clearly motivated by the perception that they are enjoyable and inherently rewarding. Persuading people not to smoke or use illicit drugs, to drink in moderation and to refrain from unprotected sex is laudable from a rational and from a public health perspective. However, this intention is actively resisted by many powerful factors. The effectiveness of prevention and harm minimization strategies is discussed in Chapter 12. It is emphasized that both legal and illegal drug use are influenced by a bewildering constellation of factors. Different people are influenced by different factors at various stages of their drinking or other drug-using careers. It is probable that other forms of human activity, such as sexual behaviour, are also influenced by a variety of complicated and sometimes contradictory forces. These must be taken into account when attempting to understand these behaviours or when attempting to modify them.

2 Drinking habits

Most of this book is about 'psychoactive' drugs. These are substances which have an effect upon the mental state and thereby the mood. Detailed accounts of drug effects are available elsewhere (e.g. Jacobs and Fehr 1987; Plant 1987; Royal College of Psychiatrists 1986). The major types of psychoactive drugs are depressants, stimulants and hallucinogens. Some drugs (such as cannabis) have both depressant and hallucinogenic properties. Others, such as Ecstasy, have both stimulant and hallucinogenic effects. Alcohol is primarily a depressant. It produces a slowing of the rate of activity of the central nervous system, which as with other depressants, may induce a feeling of relaxation. To the drinker the feeling is of increased confidence and enjoyment in social situations, thus the mistaken belief that alcohol is a stimulant. Conversely tobacco, which really is a stimulant, is frequently assumed to be a depressant due to its effect of reducing tension. It is not pejorative to classify alcohol as a 'drug'. Drugs in themselves are not intrinsically good or bad, legal or illegal. In the public mind the word 'drug' is often perceived as referring solely to illicit substances. Such limitation is technically incorrect. Alcohol use is both legal and widely approved in most countries. It is, nevertheless, a drug. As the Royal College of Psychiatrists (1986) has noted, it is 'Our Favourite Drug'.

This book is concerned with young people. Even so, the use of alcohol, tobacco and illicit drugs by the young can be realistically appreciated only if placed in the more general context of the use (and misuse) of these substances by society at large. Accordingly a brief review is presented in this chapter of general patterns for alcohol use during recent years.

Because alcohol is both legal and widely used there is information available about the quantities that are produced under legal conditions. In some countries, such as Norway, illicit alcohol production is believed to be extensive. In addition, in some developing countries a considerable amount of alcohol is home produced and is not included in 'official

Table 2.1 National alcohol consumption (1970–88)

Countries	Litres per head of 100% alcohol								
	1970	1975	1980	1983	1984	1985	1986	1987	1988
European Community									
Belgium	9.0	10.1	10.9	10.8	10.6	10.5	10.2	10.7	10.1
Denmark	–	6.9	10.6	10.4	10.6	10.4	10.5	10.3	10.0
France	17.4	17.2	15.8	14.8	14.1	13.9	13.5	13.2	13.3
Greece (beer and wine)	5.3	5.3	6.7	6.8	6.8	6.8	6.2	5.7	5.8
Ireland, Rep. of (inc. cider)	–	5.9	7.7	7.3	6.1	6.2	6.5	6.2	5.7
Italy	14.1	13.2	12.3	11.7	11.5	11.0	9.9	9.3	8.9
Luxembourg	11.8	12.7	13.0	14.1	14.9	14.3	14.1	14.3	14.2
Netherlands	5.6	8.8	8.8	8.9	8.6	8.5	8.5	8.3	8.3
Portugal	9.8	13.1	10.8	13.1	12.4	12.8	11.0	10.5	10.0
Spain	12.0	13.8	13.4	12.5	11.2	11.5	11.5	12.5	11.3
UK	5.3	6.8	7.2	6.9	7.1	7.2	7.2	7.2	7.4
West Germany	12.1	13.2	13.4	13.1	12.6	12.7	12.4	12.0	12.0
Rest of Europe									
Austria	10.3	10.8	10.8	11.3	11.0	11.0	11.0	11.2	11.4
Bulgaria	6.7	8.2	8.7	8.8	9.2	8.8	9.3	8.9	8.8
Czechoslovakia	9.3	10.1	10.5	10.5	10.3	10.1	9.8	9.8	9.7
East Germany	7.5	9.7	12.0	12.6	12.2	12.3	12.5	12.7	13.0
Finland	4.3	5.9	6.1	6.1	6.2	6.3	6.7	6.9	6.7
Hungary	9.1	10.1	11.8	11.3	11.7	11.6	11.4	10.7	10.5
Iceland	3.1	3.4	3.7	3.8	4.0	4.0	4.0	4.0	4.2
Norway	3.6	4.3	4.6	3.8	4.0	4.2	4.2	4.4	4.3
Poland	5.1	6.9	8.4	6.1	6.7	6.7	6.8	6.9	6.7

Romania	–	6.1	7.6	7.9	7.7	7.7	7.7	7.7	7.6
Sweden	5.8	6.4	5.6	5.2	5.2	5.3	5.5	5.4	5.5
Switzerland	10.3	10.2	10.6	10.8	10.9	10.9	10.8	10.8	10.9
USSR	6.8	6.8	8.8	8.3	8.4	7.2	4.4	3.2	3.6
Yugoslavia	7.9	8.1	7.8	8.1	8.1	7.7	8.1	7.8	6.9
Africa									
South Africa	3.0	3.6	3.8	4.3	4.3	4.2	4.2	4.5	4.5
Asia									
Japan (includes sake)	4.8	5.4	5.6	6.1	5.9	6.1	6.1	6.2	6.6
Philippines	–	–	4.0	4.2	4.0	3.7	3.8	–	–
Australasia									
Australia	8.0	9.4	9.5	9.4	9.2	9.3	9.4	9.0	9.1
New Zealand	6.4	7.9	8.2	7.8	8.1	7.9	8.0	8.2	7.8
North America									
Canada	6.4	8.3	8.8	8.2	8.0	8.0	7.8	7.9	7.7
USA	7.2	8.0	8.2	8.1	7.9	7.8	7.7	7.6	7.3
Central and South America									
Argentina	–	–	11.5	10.1	9.6	8.9	9.1	8.9	8.1
Brazil (beer and wine)	0.7	1.0	1.3	1.4	1.4	1.4	1.9	1.9	1.8
Chile (beer and wine)	5.8	5.4	6.5	5.4	5.5	5.6	5.6	5.2	5.2
Colombia (beer only)	1.7	1.6	2.2	2.6	2.5	2.8	2.7	2.8	2.6
Cuba (beer only)	0.8	1.1	1.2	1.3	1.3	1.3	1.4	1.4	1.6
Mexico	2.2	2.4	2.9	2.6	2.6	2.8	2.6	2.9	2.8
Peru	2.4	3.5	4.6	4.5	4.4	4.6	4.9	2.2	2.2
Venezuela (beer and wine)	–	2.5	3.8	3.6	3.6	3.1	3.1	3.7	3.8

Unless otherwise stated these figures include beer, wine and spirits and exclude cider.
The figures for Luxembourg have attempted to overcome the distortion due to cross-border trading.
Source: Brewers' Society 1990:74

statistics'. Even so, the latter provide an invaluable guide to both national and temporal patterns of alcohol consumption. These are illustrated by Table 2.1.

As this table shows, there has been considerable national variation in relation to both per capita levels of alcohol consumption and consumption trends over time. The United Kingdom is a medium level country in relation to alcohol consumption. In 1988 nine other EEC countries (excluding Greece, where data are incomplete) recorded higher levels of per capita alcohol consumption than the United Kingdom (UK). Alcohol consumption in the UK was approximately half that in France and Luxembourg and was similar to that in the USA, Canada and New Zealand. As Table 2.1 shows, over the period 1970–88 there were some marked differences in national consumption trends. Alcohol consumption declined in France, Italy and the USSR, and remained relatively stable in Belgium, West Germany and Sweden. In contrast, alcohol consumption rose in the Netherlands, South Africa and Japan. Alcohol consumption in the UK remained virtually unchanged between 1980 and 1988. It should be noted that national per capita alcohol consumption is not a perfect guide to drinking patterns. There are substantial national (and regional) variations in the proportions of males and females who drink and who abstain. Alcohol consumption is also influenced by a host of social and cultural factors (e.g. Pittman and Snyder 1962). Most people in Britain drink alcoholic beverages, if only occasionally. Recent surveys indicate that in England, Wales and Scotland approximately 5–7 per cent of men and 8–12 per cent of women report not having consumed alcohol in the previous year (e.g. Dight 1976; Breeze 1985a, 1985b; Goddard and Ikin 1988; Foster, Wilmot and Dobbs 1990).

A different pattern is evident in Northern Ireland, where over half the women and nearly a third of men have been found to be complete abstainers (Wilson 1980a).

Between the end of the Second World War and 1979 per capita alcohol consumption in the United Kingdom almost doubled. Since then it has declined slightly and has levelled out. This is illustrated by Figure 2.1.

As this figure shows, alcohol consumption was markedly higher at the beginning of the twentieth century than it has been since. This is important to note in view of recent mass media suggestions that alcohol consumption has reached unprecedented levels.

Detailed surveys of alcohol consumption in Britain have been conducted routinely during the past two decades. These uniformly indicate, as do surveys from other countries, that males are less likely than females to be abstainers and that males also generally consume larger quantities than females. This is illustrated by Table 2.2.

It has been suggested that drinking habits vary greatly in different parts of the United Kingdom. The conventional view, supported by some survey

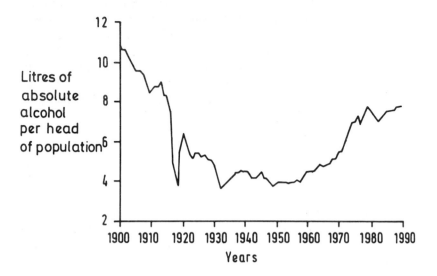

Figure 2.1 Per capita alcohol consumption in the United Kingdom (1900–89)
Source: Thurman 1991

Table 2.2 Weekly alcohol consumption amongst males and females in Britain (1988)

Consumption level (units per week) *	Persons aged 18 or over **	
	Males %	Females %
Non-drinkers	7	12
Less than 1 unit	10	24
1–10	35	40
11–21	22	14
22–35	13	7
36 50	7	2
51+	7	2
Total	101	101

* A unit is equivalent to a public house measure of spirits or to half a pint of normal strength beer, lager, stout or cider or to a single glass of wine.
** Note base total includes 102 men and 92 women for whom consumption level could not be calculated.
Source: Foster *et al.* 1990: 128

data (e.g. Office of Population Censuses and Surveys 1980) is that 'heavy drinking' is more commonplace in Scotland, Wales and Northern England than in the Midlands or South of England. Considerable attention has been paid to such regional divisions. Surveys indicate that variations in local drinking habits do exist and that some of these are quite marked (Plant and Pirie 1979; Wilson 1980a, 1980b; Crawford *et al.* 1984; Breeze 1985b). The General Household Survey for 1988 examined regional variations in self-reported alcohol consumption in Britain. This study indicated that amongst males aged 16 and over, the lowest proportions of non-drinkers (5 per cent) were in East Anglia and the Outer Metropolitan area of London. The highest proportions of non-drinkers (9 per cent) were in Greater London and Scotland. Amongst females the lowest proportions of non-drinkers were in the 'Outer South East' of England (9 per cent) and the Outer Metropolitan area (8 per cent). The highest proportions of female non-drinkers, were in Greater London (14 per cent) and Scotland (18 per cent). Fifteen per cent of females in Wales were also found to be non-drinkers. Marked regional differences were also found in relation to the proportions of males and females who had consumed 'high' levels of alcohol. These differences are shown in Table 2.3.

Table 2.3 Regional variations in 'high' levels of alcohol consumption by males and females

Region	Males (22 units or more per week) %	Females (15 units or more per week) %
North	31	10
Yorkshire and Humberside	28	11
North West	31	12
East Midlands	29	11
West Midlands	29	11
East Anglia	21	7
South East:		
Greater London	26	10
Outer Metropolitan Area	25	11
Outer South East	23	13
Total	25	11
South West	21	11
Wales	28	8
Scotland	22	7
Great Britain	26	10

Source: Foster *et al.* 1990: 143

As shown by Table 2.3, the proportions of males aged 16 or over who had reportedly consumed at least twenty-two units per week ranged from 21 per cent in East Anglia and the South West to 31 per cent in the North and North West of England. Amongst females the proportions who had consumed at least fifteen units per week ranged from 7 per cent in East Anglia and Scotland to 12 per cent in North West England and 13 per cent the Outer South East of England.

LEARNING ABOUT ALCOHOL

As the preceding pages indicate, alcohol is used by the great majority of people in Britain as well as by most of those in Northern Ireland. Young people in Britain are raised in a 'wet' culture. This means a social context in which drinking is both widely practised and generally regarded as a legitimate and enjoyable activity. The legal and social context of drinking is, in important respects, quite different from that of illicit drug use. The latter is both illegal and also widely regarded as socially unacceptable. Most young people in Britain have parents who drink and come into contact with other adults who mainly drink. In spite of this it needs to be emphasized that children raised in some areas (such as parts of the Scottish Highlands and Islands) or those born to Muslim parents may have quite different early learning experiences about alcohol.

An important study of how young children perceive alcohol was undertaken by Jahoda and Cramond (1972) in Glasgow. This investigation related to the 6–10 year age group. The researchers concluded that most of the children in this study began to learn about alcohol at home and had formed clear impressions about it well before they were old enough to attend school. Two-fifths of 6-year-olds were able to identify alcoholic beverages by smell, three-fifths could do so by the age of 10. The majority of the children in this study were also able to view drunken behaviour portrayed in a film and associate it with alcohol. Most of the children had had personal encounters with intoxicated adults. This classic study also suggested that from an early age the girls had received less adult encouragement to drink than had the boys. Jahoda and Cramond noted that as children became older they developed rather more negative attitudes towards alcohol. The researchers interpreted this as indicating that older children become aware that alcohol *misuse* is disapproved of by authority figures.[1]

Aitken (1978) examined the drinking habits of 10–14-year-olds in the Central Region of Scotland. Eighty-eight per cent of these children reported having consumed alcoholic beverages. The proportion of children who had not tried alcohol declined with age from 38 per cent at the age of 10 to only 19 per cent at the age of 14. Girls were more likely than boys to report first drinking experiences at a later age. Three-quarters of all children surveyed and 88 per cent of those who had consumed alcohol reported first drinking in their parental homes.

A fifth of the children in this study reported having been given a drink while in licensed premises. The age at which people in Britain may legally purchase alcohol or consume it in bars is 18. In addition, it is legal for people aged 16 and above to consume certain kinds of alcohol with a meal in a licensed restaurant so long as they are accompanied by people aged 18 and above. Eighteen per cent of the 10–14-year-olds reported having at some time consumed alcohol in the absence of their parents.

As noted above, Jahoda and Cramond (1972) had found that as the young children grew older they became generally rather negative in their attitudes to drinking. Similar results have recently been obtained by Fossey (1992). Aitken found that, amongst 10–14-year-olds, such negative attitudes declined with age:

> Although most of the children in each age group expressed considerable disapproval of drunkenness and spirit drinking, the severity of judgements about beer/lager and shandy/cider drinking decreased with age. For example, whereas 56 per cent of the 10 year olds said that drinking beer/ lager was 'always wrong', only 30 per cent of the 14 year olds did so.
>
> (Aitken 1978: xiv)

Aitken noted that older primary-school-aged children were able to distinguish between different types and potencies of alcoholic drinks. He also detected evidence of distinctly sexist attitudes to drinking:

> Boys tended to be less severe in their judgements of the drinking activities of boys than the girls were with respect to the drinking activities of girls. The majority of boys and girls made the same judgements about the drinking activities of the opposite sex as they did with respect to their own sex. However, those who made different judgements tended to use a 'double standard' of morality: the drinking activities of girls were judged more severely than the drinking activities of boys.
>
> (Aitken 1978: xv)

Davies and Stacey (1972) conducted another Scottish study of alcohol use amongst young people aged 14–17. This indicated that, by the age of 14, 92 per cent of boys and 85 per cent of girls had tried alcohol. By the age of 17 only 2 per cent of boys and 4 per cent of girls had not done so. The rather negative attitudes to alcohol noted by Jahoda and Cramond amongst young children were replaced by positive attitudes amongst teenagers. The latter commonly perceived drinking as a highly sociable and 'adult' activity.

Between the ages of 14 and 17 the peer group becomes the main reference group by which drinking is judged and through which it is encouraged. Most young people drink because they perceive it as a highly desirable and prestigious thing to be seen to be doing. Davies and Stacey concluded that, by the age of 17, most boys had consumed alcohol in public houses and most girls had done so in public bars or dance halls. Although drinking was commonly viewed as praiseworthy, 'heavy drinking' was regarded as unsociable and lacked such approval. In addition teenagers who did not drink were perceived as lacking in both 'toughness' and sociability.

Hawker (1978) conducted a survey of 7,278 young people aged 13–18 in England. This lent support to the conclusion that most young people become 'regular drinkers' in their early teens. The survey, like that by Davies and Stacey, indicated that teenagers are most likely to begin to drink at home and with their parents. In addition, a substantial minority reported drinking at discos and in public houses.

For most young people the family exerts a major influence on how they perceive and use alcohol. O'Connor (1978) examined the drinking habits of young people in English and Irish families. This work showed that Irish parents were more likely than English parents to discourage their children from drinking. Irish children were more likely to remain non-drinkers, but were also more likely to report adverse consequences from drinking than were their English counterparts.

Aitken and Leathar (1981) have described the results of an interesting study of adults' attitudes to drinking and smoking amongst young people. This investigation, which was conducted in Scotland, showed that most adults estimated that children begin to form a clear understanding of the distinctiveness of alcohol at or above the age of 12. As Jahoda and Cramond have demonstrated, such an understanding appeared to have developed by the age of 8. Adults were more likely to regard the youthful peer groups as more influential than parents on young people's drinking habits. Some commentators, such as Davies and Stacey (1972) and Aitken (1978), have suggested that it is a good idea for parents to introduce their children to alcohol when they are young. It is *legal* for people in Britain to consume alcohol when they are aged 5 or above. Aitken and Leathar discovered that many adults did not agree with this:

> For example, 46% said that children under 18 should not be allowed to *taste* alcoholic drinks and 63% said that children under 18 should not be allowed small drinks of their own at home with their parents. Given that most children have at least tasted alcoholic drinks in the company of parents by the age of 10 and the majority have had small drinks of their

own in the company of parents by the age of 14, these findings point to an inconsistency between actual and recommended parental practices with respect to alcohol.

(Aitken and Leathar 1981: xiv)

Aitken and Leathar also concluded that higher socio-economic status adults were inclined to give lower estimates than other adults of the age at which children have some understanding of the difference between alcoholic and non-alcoholic drinks. Higher status adults were also more likely to indicate that parents could influence their children's drinking habits. Jahoda and Cramond had not found middle-class children to be significantly different from others in relation to the development of a clear concept of alcohol. Aitken and Leathar, not surprisingly, found that adults who were themselves non-drinkers were less likely than adult drinkers to favour parents allowing their children to drink at home.

TEENAGE DRINKING

The collection of information about alcohol consumption levels amongst young people in Britain is a fairly recent activity. Hawker (1978) had concluded that it was not possible to elicit accurate consumption estimates from teenagers. Self-reports of alcohol consumption are certainly flawed. This is discussed further below. Even so, a number of studies have sought details of alcohol consumption from teenagers.

Between 1979 and 1983 a follow-up investigation was conducted of the drinking, smoking and drug-using habits of a study group of 1,036 young adults in the Lothian Region (Plant, Peck and Samuel 1985). The subjects of this study were aged 15 and 16 during its initial phase in 1979 and 1980. Only 2 per cent of both males and females reported never having consumed alcoholic beverages. Males, on average, had been a little younger than females when they had tried their first drink, 10.3 years compared with 11.6 years. Over 60 per cent of those who had consumed alcohol reported having been given their first taste by a parent, step-parent or other guardian. Over half of the study group had consumed alcohol in the past two weeks. Forty-five per cent of the boys and 31.7 per cent of the girls reported having drunk in the past week. The most common setting for drinking was the parental home. Even so, nearly a fifth reported having last drunk in a public house or hotel. As noted above, such drinking need not have been illegal since 16-year-olds are allowed to drink with meals in licensed restaurants. The alcohol consumption levels of the study group were examined by eliciting details of both the last drinking occasion and the previous week's drinking. Consumption was calculated on the basis of units of alcohol. The average levels of previous week's alcohol consumption amongst those who provided such details were 17.8 units for males and 9.2 units for females.

> Consistent with their much higher level of alcohol consumption, male respondents who reported drinking during the previous week stated that they had drunk alcohol on significantly more days than had their female counterparts: 2.3 days compared with only 1.9 days. The average maximum daily consumption reported by males during the past week was significantly higher than that reported by females: 9.1 units compared with only 4.8 units. These results show that, on average, respondents had consumed over half their total week's intake in a single day.
>
> (Plant, Peck and Samuel 1985: 27)

A general indication of the sex differences in self-reported alcohol consumption is provided by Table 2.4.

Table 2.4 Sex differences in average measures of alcohol consumption

Measures	Males (units)	Females (units)	% difference (units)
x̄ Previous week's consumption*	17.8	9.2	93.3
x̄ Maximum day's consumption in previous week *	9.1	4.8	89.6
x̄ Last occasion's consumption**	5.3	4.1	29.3

* $n = 500$
** $n = 975$
Source: Plant *et al.* 1985: 29

Overall this study lent strong support to the evidence provided by Davies and Stacey (1972), Aitken (1978) and Hawker (1978) that most teenagers are drinking on a regular basis. The respondents in the Lothian study were asked to provide details of their experience of some of the consequences of drinking. The majority, 70.4 per cent of the males and 61 per cent of the females, reported having at some time been at least mildly intoxicated. Hangovers were reported by 30.6 per cent of males and 26.3 per cent of females. Details of such adverse consequences are elaborated in Chapter 5.

The Lothian study group were sought for re-interview during 1983. They were then aged 19 and 20. By this time the cohort had left school and was widely dispersed. A total of 957 individuals, 92.4 per cent of the original respondents, were re-interviewed. The changes in self-reported alcohol consumption evident from a comparison of the two separate waves of data collection are shown in Table 2.5.

Table 2.5 Changes in self-reported alcohol consumption (1979/80–83)

Alcohol consumption measures	Males (units)	Females (units)
x̄ previous week's consumption (all respondents, drinkers only)		
1979/80	17.8	9.2
1983	23.6	9.0
% change 1979/80–83	+33.0%	−1.7%
x̄ consumption on last drinking occasion (all respondents, drinkers only)		
1979/80	4.9	4.1
1983	6.3	3.4
% change 1979/80–83	+17.0%	−17.1%

Source: Plant *et al.* 1985: 58

As this table indicates, the average level of alcohol consumed by males had increased between the ages of 15–16 and 19–20. In contrast that amongst females had *decreased*. At the age of 19–20 only 13.4 per cent of males reported not having consumed alcohol in the past week. The corresponding proportion amongst females was 26.6 per cent.

There had been a major change in the reported locations of most recent drinking since the study group members were aged 15–16. As noted above, the most commonplace venue at that age had been home. Amongst the 19–20 year olds study group the most frequently cited drinking locale was a public bar. This was reported by 50.5 per cent of males and 43.6 per cent of females. The drinking locations cited by the study group at the ages of 19–20 are shown in Table 2.6.

As this table shows, the 'home-centred' drinking amongst the study group at the age of 15–16 had been replaced by a totally different picture by the ages of 19–20. Nearly all of the respondents were still unmarried and drinking was clearly largely focused on licensed premises and places of entertainment such as clubs and discos. Consistent with this, only a minority of respondents reported having last drunk with their parents. Respondents generally reported last drinking with friends, including those of the opposite sex. Details were once more obtained about the experience of adverse consequences associated with drinking. A minority of the study

Table 2.6 Location of most recent drink

Location	Males %	Females %
Bar	50.5	43.6
Licensed club	12.5	11.0
Disco/dance	10.2	12.6
Hotel	7.7	5.8
Own home	5.8	10.6
Home of a friend	5.6	8.8
Home of a relative	1.2	1.6
Other	6.5	6.0
Total	100.0	100.0

Source: Plant et al. 1985: 59

group reported consuming relatively large amounts of alcohol. Amongst the males 8.2 per cent reported having consumed at least 51 units of alcohol in the past week. Amongst the females 2.4 per cent reported having consumed at least 31 units. The general pattern of alcohol consumption amongst this study group was similar to that for the 20–27 year age group in Scotland, England and Wales (Wilson 1980a). One of the main objectives of the Lothian-based follow-up study was to ascertain the extent to which teenagers' drinking habits change as they grow older. A comparison of alcohol consumption at the ages of 15–16 with that at 19–20 revealed only very low levels of association. It was not the case that individuals who were the heaviest drinkers at 15–16 remained the heaviest drinkers. Even so, teenagers who were heavier drinkers were more likely than others to smoke tobacco and to use illicit drugs. In addition, teenagers who were heavier drinkers at 15–16 were more likely than others to have used illicit drugs by the ages of 19–20. Ghodsian and Power (1987) examined the changing alcohol consumption of a national sample of young people in Britain between the ages of 16 and 23. This, like the Lothian study, revealed low correlations between drinking at the younger age and at 23. Even so, the authors concluded that those who drank the most at 16 were the most likely to drink heavily at the age of 23. The latter conclusion differs from that drawn by Plant, Peck and Samuel (1985). The Lothian study was continued with an additional follow-up which was carried out during 1988 and 1989. Respondents were then aged between 24 and 26 years. This phase of the study showed that drinking habits at this age bore very little resemblance to those at the age of 15 or 16 (Bagnall 1991a, 1991b).

During 1986 a survey of alcohol, tobacco and illicit drug use amongst

13-year-olds in three areas of Britain was undertaken (Bagnall 1988, 1991c). These areas were Berkshire, Dyfed and the Highland Region. This study indicated that 96 per cent of respondents had consumed alcohol, with the most common ages for the first drink being 11–12 years. As noted by other researchers, parents or other adults were the most frequently cited providers of the first alcoholic drink (81 per cent). Eighty-four per cent of respondents indicated that they had consumed their first drinks at home. The overwhelming majority of these young respondents reported having consumed only modest amounts of alcohol, although 20 per cent reported having experienced a hangover.

A detailed study of adolescent drinking was carried out by Marsh, Dobbs and White (1986). This exercise related to the 13–17 age group and included surveys which were conducted in England, Wales and Scotland in 1984. A total of 4,908 teenagers completed questionnaires. This is an important study since it provided the first detailed *national* picture of drinking habits amongst teenagers.

Consistent with evidence from earlier studies, Marsh, Dobbs and White concluded that very few teenagers had never tasted alcohol and that the proportions of those who currently reported drinking increased with age. This is shown in Table 2.7.

Table 2.7 Drinkers and non-drinkers in England, Wales and Scotland (13–17 years)

Category					Age					
	13*		14		15		16		17	
	M	F	M	F	M	F	M	F	M	F
	%	%	%	%	%	%	%	%	%	%
Have never tasted alcohol										
Eng. & Wales	6	7	3	4	2	2	3	5	6	4
Scotland	9	16	4	6	2	3	9	8	4	3
Have never had a proper drink/ never drunk										
Eng. & Wales	17	20	9	10	7	9	9	10	4	8
Scotland	23	30	11	17	10	12	12	13	10	7
Drink alcohol										
Eng. & Wales	80	74	88	86	91	90	88	85	91	88
Scotland	68	54	85	78	88	85	79	79	86	89

* The '13-year-olds' included a few who were between 12 years 10 months and 13. The '15-year-olds' included a few up to 16 years 3 months.
Source: Marsh *et al.* 1986: 8–9

As this table shows, a number of national differences were evident. Scottish boys and girls appeared to be rather less likely to begin drinking early than their counterparts in England and Wales. The authors noted:

By the age of 14, however, the Scottish boys have nearly caught up with their English and Welsh peers and by the age of 15 so have most of the girls but they never do quite catch up.

(Marsh, Dobbs and White 1986: 9)

This study also indicated that Scottish teenagers drank alcohol less often than those in England and Wales. This difference did not decline with age:

Despite consistent set differences in each age group in both countries showing boys drinking more often than girls, the differences between the two countries is so great that, for example, 15 year old *girls* in England and Wales appear to drink more often than even 16 year old *boys* in Scotland.

(Marsh, Dobbs and White 1986: 9)

This study reinforced the conclusion that younger teenagers mainly drink at home, but that as they grow older public bars, clubs and discos become the most popular drinking places. Again, national differences emerged since Scottish teenagers were much less likely than those in England and Wales to report drinking in pubs or bars. Marsh, Dobbs and White commented that Scottish teenagers might be more likely than those in England and Wales to 'drink unobserved by parents or authorities'. They also noted that the Scots may have had a more restricted access to clubs and discos than teenagers in England and Wales.

As teenagers grow older, their use of public houses and other bars increases steadily. By the age of 17 most boys and girls in England and Wales and most boys in Scotland reported that they usually bought drinks for themselves in pubs or other bars. Only a minority of teenagers reported ever having been refused alcohol in licensed premises or retail outlets because of their age.

Beverage preferences were examined in some detail. This revealed that younger teenagers preferred to drink cider and shandy. Older boys favoured beer-type drinks. Girls, especially those in Scotland, generally avoided beers and increasingly consumed aperitifs or, to a lesser extent, spirits. It was noted that the latter were probably consumed in mixes or cocktails. The disparity in the beverage preferences of the genders was extremely marked and the researchers made the following comment:

It is remarkable how sex-based preferences for styles of drink emerge so strongly in people so young. It suggests, of course, that the cultural value of drinking for adolescents is very great. Drink is used not merely for pleasure, not even to create an occasion for conviviality. It confers an adult status that is at once recognisable in a way that is appropriate to their sex.

(Marsh, Dobbs and White 1986: 21)

Marsh, Dobbs and White noted that, even amongst 13-year-old boys and girls in England and Wales, 65 per cent and 47 per cent respectively reported consuming alcohol during the week in which they completed drinking diaries. The corresponding proportions amongst 13-year-olds in Scotland were 45 per cent and 32 per cent. Scottish teenagers were less likely than their English and Welsh counterparts to have drunk during the diary week. By the age of 17, 70 per cent of males and 65 per cent of females in England and Wales had drunk in the diary week compared with 65 per cent and 55 per cent of Scots. At all ages most teenagers reported drinking only modest amounts. Even so, a minority reported drinking heavily. The authors noted the need for caution when interpreting such data:

Some of these very high values undoubtedly contain a few spurious reports. A few questionnaires and diaries of this kind were taken out of the sample when returns were first inspected. Typically they were completed by younger boys each of whom claimed to be drinking sufficient alcohol in a week to prove fatal to creatures larger than themselves.

(Marsh, Dobbs and White 1986: 31)

In spite of this important limitation, Marsh, Dobbs and White concluded that some teenagers, especially boys, were really heavy drinkers:

On week days and Sundays between 1 % and 2 % claimed to have drunk more than the equivalent of five pints of beer on any single day. On Fridays this rose to 5 % and on Saturdays to 9 % among the English and Welsh adolescents and to 14 % among the Scots.

(Marsh, Dobbs and White 1986: 31)

Marsh, Dobbs and White conducted their survey in 1984. They noted that the alcohol consumption patterns reported by their 15- and 16-year-old Scottish teenagers were strikingly similar to those reported in the 1979–80 phase of the Lothian survey by Plant, Peck and Samuel (1985).

In 1988 a survey was carried out to examine the drinking habits and alcohol-related knowledge and attitudes of 6,244 pupils aged 14–16 attending a national sample of twenty-seven state secondary (high) schools in England (Plant *et al.* 1990a). Like earlier surveys, this study indicated that few teenagers have never tasted alcohol and that most of those who drank reported consuming only small quantities. Only 4 per cent reported never having tasted alcohol. Nearly 75 per cent of those surveyed reported having their first 'real' drink of alcohol between the ages of 9–14. The commonest location of reported last drink was home (36.4 per cent) although 24.5 per cent reported having last consumed alcohol in a public house, hotel, club or disco. Details were obtained of respondents' most recent drinking occasions'.

Altogether 69.6 per cent of the boys and 78.3 per cent of the girls who provided details of their most recent drinking reported having consumed no more than four units. This is equivalent to two pints of normal strength beer or lager. In contrast, 9.7 per cent of the boys and 5.1 per cent of the girls reported having last consumed 11 units or more, equivalent to at least five and a half pints of beer. The proportion of teenagers classified as 'heavy drinkers' increased markedly with age. This is shown by Table 2.8.

Table 2.8 'Heavy drinking' amongst English teenagers aged 14–16

Age	Males * %	Females ** %
14	5.4	7.1
15	10.7	10.1
16	13.5	15.5

*Male 'heavy drinkers' were defined as those consuming 11 units or more on their last drinking occasion.
**Female 'heavy drinkers' were defined as those consuming 8 units or more on their last drinking occasion.
Source: Plant *et al.* 1990a: 688

The teenagers in this survey were asked to indicate the minimum legal age at which they thought alcohol should be purchased by young adults. At present this is 18 in the United Kingdom. More than half supported a reduction in this age limit. The most popular preference (35 per cent) was for the limit to be reduced to 16. Seventy-two per cent had at some time consumed alcohol in licensed premises. Forty-three per cent of males and 34 per cent of females reported having at some time illegally purchased alcohol. Only a quarter of those surveyed reported ever having been asked their age while on licensed premises. This conclusion was consistent with that noted earlier by Marsh, Dobbs and White (1986).

The English teenagers were asked to respond to a number of questions about the relative strengths of different types of alcoholic drink. Levels of knowledge were not high. The majority wrongly reported that a single measure of whisky is stronger than a pint of beer. Over a quarter incorrectly endorsed the view that all beers are of similar strength.

During 1990 a similar survey was conducted of 14–16-year-olds in Scotland. This elicited data from 7,009 teenagers attending a national sample of twenty-three state secondary schools. Many of the findings of this study resembled those of the earlier English survey. Even so, some differences were also evident. Eighteen per cent of males and 10 per cent of females reported that on their last drinking occasion they had consumed eleven or more units. In addition, the Scottish teenagers reported drinking rather less frequently than had their counterparts in England (Plant and Foster 1991). These national differences were broadly consistent with those noted earlier by Marsh, Dobbs and White (1986).

Two additional national surveys have provided recent information about alcohol consumption patterns amongst young adults. The first of these, by Goddard and Ikin (1988) related to England and Wales. The second, by Foster, Wilmot and Dobbs (1990) related to Britain as a whole. As shown in Table 2.3, a number of distinct regional variations in drinking habits were evident. Broadly comparable variations were also noted by Goddard and Ikin. Their survey showed that amongst males and females aged 16–17 only 8 per cent were classified as 'non-drinkers'. Amongst the 18–24 group this proportion had fallen to 4 per cent of males and 6 per cent of females. Goddard and Ikin compared the average levels of alcohol consumption amongst males and females aged 18–24 in their 1987 study with comparable individuals surveyed by Wilson (1980b) during 1978. During this period UK per capita alcohol consumption, as indicated by Figure 2.1, had changed little, declining slightly from 7.3 litres to 7.2 litres. This comparison revealed that the average previous week's alcohol consumption amongst young men had *fallen* from 26 units in 1978 to 21.4 units in 1987. Amongst young women a small fall had occurred, from 8.9 units to 8 units. The authors also, interestingly, reported that males and females who had been aged 18–24 in 1978 had also reduced their alcohol consumption between 1978 and 1987.

The Target Group Index (TGI) of the British Market Research Bureau is an annual survey of 25,000 people. This exercise examines the purchase and use of a large number of items, including alcoholic drinks. Duffy (1991) has reviewed TGI alcohol consumption data for Britain 1978–89. This analysis indicated that amongst the 15–19 age group, both for males and females, the frequency of drinking had remained little changed over this twelve-year period.

Foster, Wilmot and Dobbs (1990) classified 7 per cent of males and 9 per cent of females aged 16–24 as 'non-drinkers'. They also concluded that young men and women who were living with their parents were twice as likely as other young adults to be classified as non-drinkers. Conversely, males (but not females) were more likely to be classified as fairly–very high alcohol consumers if they were living apart from their parents.

The Health Education Authority commissioned two studies of health and lifestyles amongst young people in England. The first of these related to the 9–15 age range, the second to those 16–19 years old. These studies produced results generally consistent with the other evidence cited in this chapter. Amongst those aged 9–15 those who were regular drinkers were more likely than others to be regular smokers and to have used illicit drugs (Health Education Authority 1989). The survey of 16–19-year-olds indicated that 50 per cent of males and 44 per cent of females had at some time chosen to have a 'low alcohol' drink rather than a 'conventional' alcoholic beverage. Those from high socio-economic backgrounds were more likely than those from lower socio-economic backgrounds to have consumed low alcohol drinks. Respondents in the North of England were less likely than those elsewhere to have consumed low alcohol drinks. This study indicated that most young drinkers had experienced adverse consequences from drinking, such as hangovers. Even so knowledge of the unit content of specific drinks and of recommended 'safe limits' was poor (Health Education Authority 1990).

A recent survey of drinking habits in England and Wales provided details of the proportions of young people who consumed more than 21 units per week (males) or 14 units per week (females). Amongst those aged 16–17 these proportions were 13 per cent (males) and 8 per cent (females). Amongst those aged 18–24 the corresponding proportion rose to 33 per cent of males and 10 per cent of females. The same study also indicated which proportions of young people had consumed at least 50 units per week (males) and 35 units per week (females). Amongst those aged 16–17, 2 per cent of males and 1 per cent of females had consumed such large amounts. Amongst those aged 18–24 the corresponding proportions were 10 per cent (males) and 3 per cent (females) (Goddard 1991).

In summary, it appears that most British children become aware of alcohol at a young age. Initial, rather negative perceptions are increasingly replaced during the teenage years by a positive orientation to alcohol which is reinforced by peers and which fosters and accompanies widespread and regular drinking. The overwhelming majority of teenagers do drink and many drink in licensed premises before they are legally permitted to do so. As noted above, British surveys did not routinely collect alcohol consumption data before the 1970s. Due to this only a limited basis exists for monitoring recent trends in youthful alcohol use. The comparisons which are possible, for example between data collected, firstly, by Plant, Peck and

Samuel (1985) and Marsh, Dobbs and White (1986) and, secondly, by Wilson (1980b) and by Goddard and Ikin (1988), do not indicate any recent increase in youthful alcohol consumption levels. On the contrary, the first comparison (1979/80–4) suggested stability and the second (1978–87) indicated a *decline* in alcohol consumption levels. As indicated by Figure 2.1, UK alcohol consumption has generally been far lower than at the beginning of this century. In addition, UK alcohol consumption has been relatively stable since the early 1980s, although it has been increasing slightly.

A substantial minority of teenagers do drink heavily and this proportion appears to grow amongst older teenagers and those in their early twenties. The extent of alcohol misuse and the adverse consequences of drinking are discussed in Chapter 5. Alcohol is by far the most widely used of the psychoactive drugs considered in this book. It is associated with much less health damage than tobacco but with far more than the less widely used illicit drugs. The very popularity of alcohol consumption has established it as a continuing source of both obvious enjoyment for most drinkers and chronic misuse by a minority of those who imbibe it.

3   Smoking habits

Tobacco, as will be elaborated in Chapter 6, is associated with vastly more health damage than any other psychoactive drug. The magnitude of tobacco-related diseases and mortality firmly establishes smoking as a very risky form of behaviour. The Royal College of Physicians described post-war trends in tobacco use in the following terms:

> Since 1950, the trend in adult cigarette consumption has been quite different in men and women. Amongst men, a slight upward trend was reversed after 1962, the year in which the first RCP Report was published. The downward trend continued till 1965 since when there has been an upward move, apart from brief falls after the 1971 Report and tax increases in 1974, 1975 and 1976. In women a steady upward trend has continued throughout the period, their average consumption rather more than doubling.
>
> (Royal College of Physicians 1977: 16)

In spite of the enormity of tobacco-related health damage the use of tobacco is not associated with the array of social and behavioural problems that are linked to the use of alcohol and illicit drugs. Far less research has been conducted into the 'social aspects of tobacco use' than has been carried out in relation to either alcohol or illicit drugs. For this reason this chapter and that dealing with tobacco-related harm are shorter than those related to alcohol and illicit drugs.

Between 1972 and 1982 the proportion of smokers in the adult population in Britain declined. Those aged 16 and above who smoked fell from 46 per cent to 35 per cent. Leck *et al.* (1985) reported that the proportion of adults who smoked dropped to 31 per cent by 1984. Between 1972 and 1982 the proportion of adult female smokers fell from 42 per cent to 33 per cent. The corresponding decline amongst males was from 52 per cent to 38 per cent. In 1988 only 33 per cent of men and 30 per cent of women aged 16 or above were cigarette smokers. Recent trends have been described thus:

The decrease between 1972 and 1988 in the proportion of men who smoked cigarettes was matched by an increase both in the proportion of ex-regular smokers (from 23% to 35%) and in the proportion of men who had never or only occasionally smoked cigarettes (from 25% to 35%). There was also an increase over the period in the proportion of women who were ex-regular smokers (from 10% to 19%) but the proportion of women who had never smoked cigarettes regularly remained relatively stable at about 50%. In 1988 the proportion of women who never or only occasionally smoked cigarettes was still markedly higher than that of men (51% compared with 35%).

(Foster, Wilmot and Dobbs 1990: 84)

The same authors also noted that during the period 1972–88 the prevalence of cigarette smoking had fallen amongst all age groups surveyed (16 years and older). In addition they reported that sex differences in smoking prevalence disappeared amongst the 16–19 age group by 1980 and amongst the 20–24 age group by 1988. The proportion of males aged 16–19 who smoked fell from 43 per cent in 1972 to 28 per cent in 1988. The corresponding proportions of female smokers fell from 39 per cent to 28 per cent. In 1988, 37 per cent of British males and females aged 20–24 were classified as cigarette smokers.

It is legal for people in the United Kingdom to purchase cigarettes once they are 16 years old. Foster, Wilmot and Dobbs (1990) have reported that, amongst the 16–17 age group, only 23 per cent of males and 20 per cent of females smoked cigarettes. However, these authors concluded that their results were probably underestimates.

Goddard has described an important study in *Why Children Start Smoking* (1990). As the book's title indicates, this exercise attempted to investigate the reasons for youthful smoking in face of widespread information that this form of behaviour is extremely dangerous. Goddard noted that the Theory of Reasoned Action described by Fishbein and Ajzen (1975) was consistent with the cessation of smoking by adults. This theory, like that of deviant behaviours propounded by Matza (1964, 1969), suggested that the adoption of a behaviour was likely to be preceded by attitude change. This view has been supported in relation to the use by young people of illicit drugs (Plant 1975). Goddard reported that first smoking experiences could, accordingly, be expected to be preceded by the formation of positive attitudes to smoking.

Her study involved a survey of pupils aged 11–19 in a sample of secondary (high) schools in England and Wales. This survey suggested that the adoption of smoking by children was, in Goddard's words, 'seldom a distinct event' and was 'more erratic' than smoking amongst adults.

Goddard concluded that the most important factors which fostered youthful tobacco smoking were the following:

- being a girl
- having brothers or sisters who smoke
- having parents who smoke
- living with a lone parent
- having relatively less negative views about smoking
- not intending to stay on in full-time education after 16
- thinking that they might be a smoker in the future.

(Goddard 1990: ix)

It was reported that most children in the age range 11–15 do not smoke regularly and that for most of those who do smoke this is 'opportunistic'. This was illustrated with reference to the availability of ways to purchase cigarettes and/or of friends who provide cigarettes. No general movement from occasional to heavy smoking was noted, even though some children did progress in this manner. She concluded that young people, including smokers, had generally very negative attitudes to smoking. In addition, the evidence of this study did not support the theories of Matza and Fishbein and Ajzen that attitude changes precede the adoption of a new behaviour.

Goddard noted that both the attitudes and behaviours of her sample of children were unstable over time.

The impression gained from the data is that many pupils did not have developed and consistent views about the particular consequences of smoking about which they were asked, and so answered the questions in a general way which reflected their overall feelings about smoking. The relatively small number of children who expressed views markedly different from those of their peers were more likely to change them subsequently – this lends support to the idea that they had not thought them out fully, or were more likely to succumb to peer pressure.

(Goddard 1990: 67)

Another major study by Goddard (1989) examined the smoking habits of secondary school pupils in England during 1988. This exercise was the fourth national study of smoking amongst teenagers carried out for the Department of Health (Dobbs and Marsh 1983, 1985; Goddard and Ikin 1987). The 1988 survey confirmed that smoking amongst boys had declined since the earlier studies. No significant change, however, was evident amongst girls, even though the proportion of smokers had declined.

Between 1982 and 1988 the proportion of boys who smoked regularly or occasionally fell from 18 per cent to 10–13 per cent. The corresponding proportions amongst girls fell from 20 per cent to 10–17 per cent. These percentages relate to test and control groups. Boys who smoked regularly had smoked more cigarettes than girls who smoked regularly (a mean of 52 in the past week compared with a mean of 44). The highest proportions of regular smokers were resident in the South of England and Greater London. The proportion of teenagers who smoked increased with age from very few at the age of 11 years to 16–18 per cent of boys and 17–27 per cent of girls aged 15. Goddard concluded that children were markedly more likely to smoke if other family members also did so. She noted:

> Brothers and sisters appeared to have more influence in this respect than did parents – pupils with brothers and sisters who smoked were much more likely than other pupils to be smokers themselves, irrespective of the smoking behaviour of their parents. Overall, those who had at least one brother or sister who smoked were five times as likely to be smokers themselves as were those who did not.
>
> (Goddard 1989: vii)

Goddard reported that approximately a quarter of the 11–15-year-olds surveyed had attempted to purchase cigarettes from shops in the previous year. Such purchase is illegal for those under the age of 16. Only 8 per cent had been refused by shopkeepers on their last attempt to buy cigarettes.

In the previous chapter it was noted that young people who drink heavily have also been reported to be especially likely to smoke and to use illicit drugs. Consistent with this, Goddard noted that at each age from 11–15 frequent drinkers were far more likely than other children to have smoked tobacco.

Sussnam *et al.* (1989) examined the relationship between the use of smokeless tobacco and other behaviours amongst seventh grade students in Los Angeles. This study showed that 'risk-taking' was associated with such tobacco use. Sports participation was associated with smokeless tobacco use only amongst one cohort of females but not at all amongst males. The authors inferred from their results that smokeless tobacco was particularly likely to have been used by males who enjoyed taking risks, and who smoked cigarettes and drank alcohol.

Swadi (1989) has reported that adolescent truancy from school was strongly associated with daily tobacco smoking and the use of solvents. He further concluded that truanting boys were especially likely to use illicit drugs, while girls who truant are more likely to drink alcohol. Swadi suggested that preventing or reducing truancy might reduce the risks of involvement with drug use. He also noted a closer relationship between truancy and illicit drug use than between truancy and alcohol consumption.

Foster, Wilmot and Dobbs (1990) found that, amongst those aged 16–24, individuals who lived with their parents were less likely to smoke than were those living away from their parental homes. In addition, young adults whose parents both smoked were markedly more likely to smoke themselves:

Young women were more likely to smoke (43%) than young men (38%) if both their parents were smokers but were less likely to do so if neither parent smoked (17% compared with 23%) or if one parent smoked (27% compared with 32%).

(Foster, Wilmot and Dobbs 1990: 91)

Cigarette smoking is inversely related to socio-economic status and with educational level. Those with non-manual jobs and/or higher educational qualifications are those least likely to smoke. Only 18 per cent of males and 12 per cent of females with degrees were smokers compared to 44 per cent and 42 per cent respectively of those without formal educational qualifications.

The encouraging decline in the prevalence of smoking has been accompanied by a fall in the average weekly cigarette consumption of young males who continue to smoke. Amongst males in the age group 16–19 this fell from 102 cigarettes per week in 1972 to eighty-four cigarettes per week in 1988. This decline contrasted with a slight *increase* in the weekly number of cigarettes smoked by young female smokers (from seventy-six to seventy-nine). In addition, older male smokers also slightly *increased* their cigarette consumption between 1972 and 1988.

As noted above, 28 per cent of males and females in the 16–19 age group were classified as cigarette smokers in 1988. Twenty-one per cent of young males smoked fewer than twenty cigarettes per day, while 6 per cent smoked twenty or more. Amongst young females 23 per cent smoked fewer than twenty cigarettes per day and 5 per cent smoked twenty cigarettes or more.

Over the period 1974–88 a number of marked geographical variations in smoking prevalence were evident. These are elaborated in Table 3.1.

As this table indicates, the fall in the prevalence of cigarette smoking has been general. Even so, the fall has not been so marked in Scotland and the North of England. This probably reflects a variety of factors, including the socio-economic composition of the populations in different areas. Comparable regional differences had been reported earlier by Bostock and Davies (1979).

A recent survey of teenage smoking in England by MORI (1990) indicates that by the age of 9, 8 per cent of children had tried smoking and that this proportion rose to 38 per cent at 13 and 61 per cent at 15. Girls were more likely to smoke than boys, 24 per cent and 17 per cent respectively by the age of 15. This study also indicated that the highest rates of smoking

Table 3.1 Prevalence of cigarette smoking by region (1974 and 1988)

Region	1974 % (over 16s)	1988 % (over 16s)
England		
North	46	36
Yorkshire and Humberside	43	32
North West	48	33
East Midlands	44	32
West Midlands	45	29
East Anglia	39	29
Greater London	No data	34
Outer Metropolitan	46	29
Outer South East	No data	28
South West	41	28
Wales	46	31
Scotland	48	37
Great Britain	45	32

Source: Foster *et al.* 1990: 115

amongst teenagers were evident in South East England and in London. In contrast, rates in the North, East Anglia and the East Midlands were well below the national average. Children who had at least one parent who smoked were twice as likely as others to become regular smokers. Three-quarters of regular smokers reported that most of their friends smoked in contrast to only 3 per cent of teenagers who did not smoke.

Most of the tobacco in Britain is consumed in the form of cigarettes. In 1988, 79 per cent of male cigarette smokers and 96 per cent of female cigarette smokers used mainly filter cigarettes. In addition, 47 per cent of those who smoked manufactured cigarettes used 'low to middle tar' varieties. Amongst people aged 16–19 females reported only cigarette smoking, while 1 per cent of males reported smoking a pipe and 2 per cent reported smoking cigars (Foster, Wilmot and Dobbs 1990).

As noted earlier, tobacco is associated with vastly more health damage than the illicit drugs or even alcohol. At the time of writing tobacco is also associated with more deaths than AIDS.

Accordingly, it is good to conclude from available evidence that tobacco use has been declining in the United Kingdom. Even so, a minority of both young people and older people continue to indulge in what is obviously an extremely hazardous form of risk-taking behaviour. This persistence, over thirty years after the exposure of the dangers of tobacco smoking, high-lights the fact that the provision of information about health dangers is not, by itself, enough to eliminate risky health behaviours, even if they can be reduced.

4 Illicit drug use

The use and misuse of psychoactive drugs is inextricably associated with culture and life-styles. As noted in preceding chapters, public concern periodically becomes focused on the use of alcohol and tobacco by children, adolescents and young adults. Even so, alcohol and tobacco use or misuse are seldom claimed to be the monopoly of the young. Indeed, evidence emphasizes that the middle-aged and even the elderly are as likely to misuse alcohol and to smoke tobacco as are the young. In contrast, the use of illicit drugs, such as cannabis, LSD, cocaine and the opiates, is widely perceived as being particularly a youthful form of behaviour.

For the purposes of this book 'illicit drugs' are defined as substances covered by the Misuse of Drugs Act (1971) and by related legislation. This definition encompasses substances such as cocaine, opium, heroin, methadone, morphine, LSD, mescaline, psilocybin, cannabis, amphetamines, 'angel dust' and a variety of tranquillizers (Plant 1987: 47–52). Glues and solvents, though not covered by the Misuse of Drugs Act, are sometimes misused and are regarded in this text as being closely allied with 'illicit drugs'. 'Prescribed drugs' are taken to be substances which are normally available on prescription but which are also used on a non-prescription basis (on the black market). These include opiate-like drugs, amphetamines and a variety of tranquillizers.

As emphasized in preceding chapters, drug use is a popular human activity. In most countries both alcohol and tobacco use are legal and socially approved. The use of 'illicit drugs' by definition is illegal. It is also widely perceived as socially unacceptable and dangerous. During the eighteenth and nineteenth centuries opium was legal and widely used in Britain (Berridge and Edwards 1981). During the twentieth century other, newer drugs have gained popularity for recreational purposes and determined international action has been taken to restrict the production, distribution and use of such drugs. The latter are now subject to rigid control policies in many countries.

Opium and cocaine were in circulation in Britain during the early part of this century. In 1916 the Commissioner of Police for the Metropolis of London reported on cocaine trafficking. Jeffrey noted that:

Nevertheless abuse of cocaine continued to be a problem in London for years, as shown by the fact that in 1921, the first year of operation of the Dangerous Drugs Act (1920), out of 67 prosecutions in respect of drugs other than opium, 58 related to cocaine.

(Jeffrey 1970: 60)

Between the 1920s and the 1960s illicit drug use provoked little concern in Britain. The so-called 'British System' of managing drug dependence was established in 1926. This emphasized drug dependence as a clinical problem and facilitated the provision of legal drug supplies to dependent individuals. Between 1935 and 1955 the number of people recorded as dependent fell from 700 to fewer than 400.

After the Second World War there was evidence of a rise in the re-creational use of both cannabis and heroin. The latter constituted a cause for serious concern, accentuated by the fact that some heroin users were clearly eager to encourage others to join in their activities. An initial report by an official body, the Brain Committee, was reassuring. However, a second report, published in 1965, concluded that there was a marked growth in drug misuse. Since that date it has been widely acknowledged that drug misuse has indeed become a widespread, chronic problem. This has led to the introduction of new legislation and a variety of policy recommendations, the most recent of which also relate to HIV infection (e.g. Plant 1987; Advisory Council on the Misuse of Drugs 1982, 1984, 1988, 1989).

The rise of concern about drug use and, in particular, alarm at the prospect of the 'proselytizing' heroin user coincided with the development, both in Britain and elsewhere, of a distinctive youth culture. This culture, with its characteristic fashions of dress, music, ideology and behaviour, has been closely involved with both the initial and the continued use of illicit drugs. As noted by Young (1971), Goode (1970, 1972) and several other authors, the use of cannabis and other illicit substances was merely part of a life-style that encompassed hedonism, experience-seeking and a rejection of 'straight' or 'conventional values'. Youth culture, with its mods, rockers, Hell's Angels, hippies, punks and acid rockers, has provided an enduring source of both fascination and alarm. As vividly described by Cohen (1972), much of the mass media portrayal of the real and imagined excesses of young people has been exaggerated and distorted. Such alarm has been aptly named as 'moral panic'. Underlying such panics has been the fact that young people are often more affluent and mature than were their forebears.

In addition, 'youth culture' has become the popular culture not just of teenagers, but that of younger people and their parents.

Surveys of self-reported drug use do not have a long tradition in Britain. The great majority of such studies have been conducted since 1970. Surveys provide a valuable guide to the extent of drug use. Even so, most have been small-scale and confined to atypical study groups. In addition, as noted in Chapter 2, survey results are clearly distorted by exaggeration, under-reporting, non-contact and refusal to co-operate. Accordingly, it is emphasized that survey data should be interpreted with caution.

Binnie and Murdock (1969) conducted one of the earliest British drug surveys. This related to higher education students in Leicester. The study showed that 9 per cent of those surveyed reported having at some time used some form of illicit drug. A survey of people aged 17–24 in Cheltenham indicated that a fifth had used cannabis, LSD or amphetamines (Plant 1973).

A study of medical students in Glasgow indicated that 14 per cent had used illicit drugs (McKay, Hawthorne and McCartney 1973). A second Glaswegian study examined drug use amongst school pupils, students, casualty unit patients and people attending clinics for sexually transmitted diseases. Those included in this investigation were aged 16–24. This study indicated that 31 per cent of those surveyed had used illicit drugs (Fish *et al.* 1974). Another university-based study by Kosviner and Hawks (1977) revealed that a third of the study group in two colleges had used illicit drugs. As noted above, few 'national' surveys of drug use in Britain have been conducted. The British Crime Survey was carried out in 1981. This included questions about self-reported cannabis use but did not examine the use of other types of drug. This study indicated that 16 per cent of those aged 20–24 in England and Wales had used cannabis and that the corresponding proportion in Scotland was 19 per cent (Chambers and Tombs 1984; Mott 1989).

During 1982 the *Daily Mail* commissioned a rare national survey of drug use. Unlike the British Crime Survey this was not confined to cannabis. The *Daily Mail* survey related to the 15–21 age group. The results of this study are shown in Table 4.1.

As this table indicates, cannabis was the most widely used drug. Self-reported levels of drug use varied markedly in different areas of Britain. The use of barbiturates, LSD, heroin and cocaine was highest in Scotland. It must be noted that very few Scottish respondents were included in this survey, so such percentages may be misleading. With the exception of Scotland, heroin and cocaine use was reported by only a very small minority of respondents.

Williams (1986) has described the results of a survey of 2,417 secondary school and college students in England and Wales. This study indicated that

Table 4.1 Regional patterns of self-reported illicit drug use amongst people aged 15–21

Drugs ever used	Scotland	North of England	Midlands, East Anglia, Wales	South of England (Excluding London)	London
	(n = 57*) %	(n = 447*) %	(n = 338*) %	(n =330*) %	(n = 153*) %
Cannabis	21	15	16	13	28
Amphetamines	8	4	6	3	10
Glues	2	5	1	2	4
Barbiturate	16	2	4	2	3
LSD	8	3	4	2	3
Heroin	7	+**	1	1	1
Cocaine	3	1	1	1	1

* Weighted total
** Less than 0.5 per cent
Source: NOP Market Research Ltd 1982

17 per cent had at some time used cannabis, 6 per cent had used glues or solvents and 2 per cent had used heroin.

Several studies have examined self-reported drug use in specific areas. These support the conclusion of the British Crime Survey and that conducted for the *Daily Mail* that there are marked regional variations in drug use.

Pritchard *et al.* (1986) conducted a survey of self-reported drug use amongst 808 teenagers in Bournemouth and Southampton. The individuals surveyed were aged 14–16. A total of 19 per cent of respondents reported having used illicit drugs or solvents. The most commonly used substances were cannabis, glue, gas, typewriter fluid and amphetamines. Levels of self-reported drug use did not differ significantly between teenagers in the two cities. Eleven per cent of the teenagers surveyed were classified as 'Drug Abusers', having used 'cannabis or other non-hallucinogens'. (Some commentators would categorize cannabis as a hallucinogen.) Four per cent of the study group were classified as a 'Serious Abuse' group, having reportedly used drugs such as heroin, cocaine, LSD, amphetamines, other hallucinogens as well as cannabis and solvents. The authors noted that teenagers classified as 'abusers' were especially likely to have unemployed fathers and to have older siblings. The 'abusers' were more likely than other teenagers to smoke tobacco and to be classified as 'under-aged drinkers'. Truancy from school was more commonplace amongst the abusers than amongst other teenagers, as were self-reported involvement in fighting and vandalism.

As noted in Chapter 2, between 1979 and 1988 a follow-up study monitored the drinking, smoking and illicit drug use of a study group of young people in the Lothian Region in South Central Scotland. These individuals were aged 15 and 16 in 1979. At the beginning of the study 15 per cent of males and 11 per cent of females reported having used some form of illicit drug. Five years later drug experience had risen to 37 per cent of males and 23 per cent of females (Plant, Peck and Samuel 1985). Cannabis was by far the most commonly used drug and fewer than 1 per cent of the study group reported having ever used heroin.

The same study group was sought for re-interview during 1988 and 1989. Three-quarters of its members were successfully contacted. Twenty-nine per cent of both males and females (then aged 25 and 26) recalled having at some time used illicit drugs. Cannabis was still overwhelmingly the most commonly used substance, 22 per cent, use of amphetamines was reported by 5 per cent and 9 per cent reported having used LSD. Cocaine had been used by 1.8 per cent and heroin by 0.5 per cent (Bagnall 1991b).

A survey of 3,333 adolescents in London state comprehensive schools has been described by Swadi (1988). This indicated that one in five of those aged 11–16 had at some time used illicit drugs or solvents. The sexes did not differ in relation to self-reported levels of drug use, except in that females were more likely than males to have used solvents and cocaine. Eight per cent of this study group had 'repeatedly' used drugs and 5.8 per cent had reportedly used drugs such as LSD, cocaine, heroin or tranquillizers.

Swadi and Zeitlin (1988) have suggested that peer influence is a major factor in encouraging adolescent drug use. They further concluded that such influence may also serve to encourage the moderation or cessation of drug use.

Parker, Bakx and Newcombe (1988) have described a detailed study of illicit drug use in the Wirral in North West England. This investigation, which was a detailed epidemiological study, included surveys of people aged 10–12, 15–16 and 16–19 respectively in schools, a Youth Training Scheme (YTS) and a college. The authors drew the following conclusions:

> The most popular illicit drug was clearly cannabis, which had been tried by three or four out of every ten of the young people surveyed. . . . The next most frequently used illicit drugs overall are magic mushrooms, tried by one in every six or seven of the respondents. However, amphetamines were more popular among the students (tried by about one in six), and was also the third most frequently used drug in YTS trainees. By contrast, solvents were used by a far higher proportion of school children

compared with the other groups. Only 2.5% of respondents reported having tried heroin. . . . and less than 1% had tried other drugs.

(Parker, Bakx and Newcombe 1988: 120)

Parker, Bakx and Newcombe noted that failure to disclose drug use might have been particularly great in relation to heroin and cocaine. Brown and Lawton (1988) conducted a survey of 1,063 pupils and students aged between 11 and 19 in Portsmouth and Havant. This study indicated that 5 per cent had used illicit drugs. Amongst those aged 11–13 only 1 per cent reported ever having used drugs (excluding solvents). Amongst those aged 14 and 15, 5 per cent had used drugs. Amongst those aged 16–19, 12 per cent reported having used drugs. The same survey indicated that glues and solvents had been used by 4 per cent of all pupils and by 7 per cent of 11-year-olds. Plant, Peck and Samuel (1985) had earlier noted that solvent use was more widely reported by people at the age of 15–16 than at the age of 19–20.

Bagnall (1988, 1991c) conducted a survey of self-reported drug use amongst 13-year-old school pupils in Berkshire, the Highlands and Dyfed. This indicated that 5 per cent had used illicit drugs.

Coggans *et al.* (1989) have described the results of a survey of self-reported drug use amongst 1,197 Scottish teenagers in twenty schools. This indicates that 22.7 per cent of respondents had used illicit drugs. The details of this are elaborated in Table 4.2.

Table 4.2 Self-reported drug use amongst Scottish teenagers

Drug	%
Cannabis	15.3
Magic mushrooms	7.3
Temazepam	6.5
LSD	5.7
Amphetamines	3.8
DF118	2.3
Barbiturates	1.7
'Other drugs'	1.7
Temgesic	1.4
Ecstasy	0.9
Cocaine	0.8
Heroin	0.7
Crack	0.2
Diconal	0.2
Astrolite	0.2

Source: Coggans *et al.* 1989: 114

The fictitious substance 'Astrolite' was included in this survey in order to indicate the extent to which teenagers might be inclined to provide misleading or fanciful answers. The fact that two of those surveyed claimed to have used this non-existent drug is a reminder of the need to treat the results of all such survey data with caution. Coggans *et al.* concluded that very few of the teenagers surveyed were frequent drug users. The proportion of those who had ever used drugs rose from 10.7 per cent amongst the youngest, aged 13, to 27.3 per cent amongst the oldest, aged 16.

Swadi (1989), describing the results of a survey of 1,232 London school pupils aged 11–17, concluded that illegal drug use and tobacco smoking and, to a lesser extent, drinking were associated with truancy. Truants were twice as likely as other adolescents to have used solvents or illicit drugs and three times more likely to have used substances such as LSD, cocaine and heroin.

Ford (1990a) conducted a survey which examined, amongst other topics, levels of self-reported drug use amongst 400 people aged 16–24 in Bristol. This indicated that 42 per cent of those surveyed had at some time used cannabis. The other drugs most widely used were 'magic mushrooms' (14 per cent), 'speed' (amphetamines) (13 per cent) and LSD (9 per cent). Five per cent reported having used cocaine and 2 per cent reported using heroin. Six respondents, 1.6 per cent, reported having at some time injected drugs.

In 1991, the Cooperative Wholesale Society produced a survey of the attitudes of children aged 9–16 to a variety of 'anti-social behaviours'. This study included 618 children in England and Scotland. This investigation revealed that 91 per cent of those surveyed classified drug taking as one of the three worst examples of anti-social behaviour. Also listed high were vandalism (90 per cent) and drunken driving (89 per cent). This negative view of illegal drug use parallels that towards drinking noted amongst young children by Jahoda and Cramond (1972).

Surveys like that illustrated by Table 4.1 suggest that marked regional variations exist in relation to levels of self-reported drug use. As noted above, surveys are certainly biased and distorted by under-reporting or exaggeration. Under-reporting is acknowledged to be a major problem in relation to surveys of alcohol use, which is legal. It is probable that such bias is an even greater limitation in relation to surveys of illicit drug use. In spite of their certain defects, surveys do provide a valuable indication of the likely approximate scale and pattern of illicit drug use. Survey data indicate that large numbers of young people do use illicit drugs. Cannabis is by far the most widely used of these substances, though several studies (e.g. Plant, Peck and Samuel 1985; Brown and Lawton 1988) indicate that glues and solvents are also used quite widely, especially by rather younger people. The widespread use of Ecstasy (MDMA) has recently been noted in several areas of the UK, notably at 'rave' parties. The use of glues and solvents by children in the 7–11 age range has been noted by several authors (e.g. Watson 1979, 1986). The use of LSD, amphetamines, cocaine, heroin and other drugs has generally been shown to be far more limited than that of cannabis and this is consistent with information related to drug offences. The latter are discussed in Chapter 7. Surveys also indicate that few people below the age of 11 use illicit drugs (with the exception of glues and solvents). Between the ages of 11 and 20 the proportion of people who have used illicit drugs increases. In some areas a quarter or a third of people have used illicit drugs by the time they have passed the age of 19.

The overall extent of illicit drug use is difficult to measure. Parker, Bakx and Newcombe (1988) have concluded that regular opioid use in the Wirral amongst people aged 16–24 was 1.8 per cent. Hartnoll *et al.* (1985) estimated that such drug use in Camden and Islington was 1.2 per cent during the period 1977–83. Robertson (1987) has noted a high level of opiate use in Muirhouse, a deprived area of Edinburgh.

Surveys consistently show that males are more likely to use illicit drugs than are females. Even so, this gender difference is not always substantial. Most people who report having used illicit drugs report having done so on only a limited number of occasions.

Most illicit drug use coincides with or follows adolescence. Smoking and drinking have a potent appeal because of their commonplace roles as hallmarks of maturity. Many young people purchase alcohol and tobacco before they are legally old enough to do so. The illegality of illicit drug use often has its own special appeal. The growth of the 'drug scene', as noted by Young (1971), was closely linked with the upsurge of youth culture and with music, behaviours and fashions designed to excite, entertain, rebel or shock. The very illegality of cannabis and other substances bestows upon them the special appeal of 'forbidden fruit'.

Drug use occurs amongst young people from all socio-economic backgrounds. Even so, there appear to be socio-economic differences in the use of heroin and of opioids. The latter has been most frequently noted amongst people living in the most deprived areas, characterized, for example, by high levels of unemployment (e.g. Pearson, Gilman and MacIver 1985; Dorn and South 1987; Parker, Bakx and Newcombe 1988). It must, however, be emphasized that the *association* between opioid use and unemployment is not a simple one. In addition, some opiate users come from affluent backgrounds.

Some individuals use illicit drugs regularly and heavily. Some people confine such drug use to a single substance such as cannabis, but many also use a wide variety of drugs, legal and illicit. The phenomenon of multiple drug use or polydrug use has been widely noted (e.g. Plant 1987; Mott

1976; Stimson 1981; Stimson and Oppenheimer 1982; Plant, Peck and Samuel 1985). There is no inevitable 'escalation' or 'progression' process involved in drug use. Drug users vary considerably and stubbornly refuse to conform to any particular stereotype. Even so, people who use illicit drugs regularly are more likely than less frequent users to use a number of different drugs, to smoke tobacco and to be relatively heavy alcohol consumers.

Several authors have concluded that truancy from school is associated with adolescent drug use. For example, Swadi (1989) reached this view on the basis of a survey of 11–17-year-olds in London. This view had earlier been reached by a variety of other authors (e.g. Jessor and Jessor 1977; Malcolm and Shephard 1978; Hundleby *et al.* 1982).

Available evidence indicates that far more people use illicit drugs than ever come to the attention of 'official agencies' in relation to 'drug problems'. Most cannabis users neither 'progress' to continued drug use nor develop drug-related adverse consequences. In spite of this, as noted by the Royal College of Psychiatrists (1987), it is probable that the overall level of illicit drug problems reflects the overall level of illicit drug use: an increase in drug use will probably be accompanied by a rise in drug misuse. The latter possibility is considered in Chapter 7.

The aetiology of drug use has been discussed in Chapter 1 and has been elaborated in Chapters 2 and 3. It is clear that, as with alcohol and tobacco, the use of illicit drugs is commonly prompted by peer pressure, by curiosity, by the enjoyment of drug effects, as well as by factors such as availability and price.

In conclusion, illicit drug use is now a commonplace phenomenon amongst young people in Britain. Available evidence suggests that, while a substantial minority of teenagers and those in their twenties have used such substances, only a small percentage do so regularly or with harmful consequences. Most of those who use illicit drugs do so for the same reasons that people drink alcohol or smoke tobacco. The commonest reasons for initiating such activity are curiosity and peer pressure, often combined with normal youthful drives towards rebellion and a wish to engage in adult or risky behaviours.

Illicit drug use amongst pre-adolescents does occur but is rather rare and appears largely to involve glues and solvents. Individuals who use illicit drugs are also likely to smoke and drink. Regular involvement with 'the drug scene' is typically characterized by multiple drug use involving both legal and illicit substances. Although survey evidence is patchy it appears that the youthful use of illicit drugs in Britain has been increasing.

5 Alcohol misuse

The misuse of alcohol by young adults, adolescents or even children periodically becomes a focus for public concern. The occasional rampages of drunken soccer 'fans' or disorderly behaviour by 'lager louts' have, on several occasions, led to intense mass media interest in heavy or problematic drinking by young people. This topic has recently been the focus of three British reports (British Medical Association 1986; Home Office 1987; Tuck 1989).

Concern about youthful alcohol misuse is by no means solely a recent phenomenon, as noted by the British Medical Association:

> Legislation at the turn of the century signalled widespread worry about the exposure of children to alcohol. The very purpose of the formation of the Band of Hope was the instruction of boys and girls on the properties of alcohol and the consequences of its consumption, and by 1901 it was reported that in the United Kingdom there were 28,894 local societies, with a total membership of 3,536,000 boys and girls.
>
> (BMA 1986: 1)

Alcohol consumption amongst young people has been considered in Chapter 2. As noted therein, general UK levels of alcohol consumption were higher at the beginning of the twentieth century than they have been in recent decades. Nevertheless, per capita alcohol consumption, having declined during the 1930s, virtually doubled between 1945 and 1979. 'Alcohol-related problems' include physical dependence or 'addiction' to alcohol, as well as a host of other adverse consequences. These encompass alcohol-related deaths, illness, social, economic and public order problems. These have been reviewed elsewhere (e.g. Royal College of Psychiatrists 1986; Royal College of Physicians 1987; Royal College of General Practitioners 1986).

In general the overall level of alcohol-related problems reflects the overall level of alcohol consumption. Rises and falls in the latter are usually accompanied by rises and falls in the former (Bruun *et al*. 1975). As alcohol consumption in the UK declined during the 1930s so too alcohol-related problems declined. During the 1950s, 1960s and 1970s the increase in per capita consumption evident both in the UK and in many other countries was accompanied by a proliferation in alcohol-related problems. As such problems became more commonplace, concern about alcohol misuse also increased. In the UK such concern, combined with obvious need, led to the creation of National Health Service clinics for problem drinkers and an impressive network of local councils specifically designed to help people with drinking problems. Alcoholics Anonymous (AA) had become established in Britain during the Second World War. AA membership expanded rapidly during the postwar decades, together with its associated fellowships Al-Anon (for the relatives of problem drinkers) and Al-Ateen (for their children).

As noted in Chapter 2, per capita alcohol consumption in the UK reached a post-war peak in 1979, declined slightly and then, recently, has been climbing slowly. It is not surprising that the general increase in alcohol problems evident while alcohol consumption was rising in earlier decades was replaced by a general levelling out as alcohol consumption stabilized.

'Alcohol misuse' amongst young people may be considered in relation to two main sources of evidence. Firstly, a considerable amount of information is available from surveys of self-reported drinking habits. Secondly, there are 'official statistics' which record details of certain indicators of alcohol misuse.

HEAVY DRINKING

There is no general definition of 'heavy drinking'. Virtually every study has used its own method of classification. This is complicated further by the fact that alcohol consumption influences people in different ways. Males and females are affected differently and specific levels of alcohol consumption exert different effects upon people of different weights. Three of the Royal Medical Colleges have recently produced reports (Royal College of Psychiatrists 1986; Royal College of General Practitioners 1986; Royal College of Physicians 1987). These identified general guidelines for low and high risk levels of alcohol consumption. 'Low risk' levels were defined as up to fourteen units per week for adult females and twenty-one units per week for males. Females who exceeded thirty-five units per week and males who exceeded fifty units were identified as consuming 'high risk' quantities of alcohol. These levels are controversial. Even so, such general guidelines serve an obvious practical purpose so long as it is understood that such guidelines are not absolute. Such general advice needs to be related to specific people such as pregnant women and to specific situations such as drinking and driving. The former is discussed in some detail in Chapter 8.

Dight (1976) had noted, from her survey of Scottish drinking habits, that 30 per cent of the alcohol consumed in a week had been imbibed by only 3 per cent of the total population. The latter were mainly males who consumed at least fifty-one units per week.

As outlined in Chapter 2, available British survey data do not indicate an increase in youthful alcohol consumption during recent years. Even so, surveys do indicate that a minority of young people consume large amounts of alcohol (e.g. Plant, Peck and Samuel 1985; Marsh, Dobbs and White 1986; Plant *et al.* 1990a; Plant and Foster 1991). Available evidence suggests that young people who are 'heavy drinkers' are more likely than others to smoke and to use illicit drugs (e.g. Plant, Peck and Samuel 1985). In addition, surveys uniformly show that individuals who drink most are, predictably, far more likely than others to experience adverse consequences related to drinking. The follow-up study by Plant, Peck and Samuel also indicated that teenagers who were heavier drinkers at the ages of 15 and 16 were subsequently more likely than other teenagers to use illicit drugs, even if they were not unduly likely to remain heavy drinkers.

Plant, Bagnall and Foster (1990) compared teenagers in England who were 'heavy drinkers' with those who drank less or who were non-drinkers. For the purpose of this analysis they classified their sample of 14–16-year-olds in relation to last drinking occasion. A division was made which singled out the 10 per cent of either sex who had reportedly consumed most alcohol. 'Heavy drinkers' were defined as males who had consumed eleven units or more and as females who had consumed eight units or more. Some differences did emerge between the heavy drinkers and other teenagers.

Female heavy drinkers were more likely to endorse the view that alcohol makes a person more alert. Male heavy drinkers were more likely than other males to agree that it is safe to drive after consuming one or two drinks. Both male and female heavy drinkers were less likely than other teenagers to agree that under-age drinking was a serious problem in Britain. The heavy drinkers were markedly more likely than other teenagers to report last consuming alcohol with friends of both sexes. The heavy drinkers were also less likely than other teenagers to have last consumed alcohol with their parents. Consistent with these differences, the heavy drinkers were also more likely to report that their most recent drink had been consumed in a public bar, hotel, club, friend's house or out of doors. Not surprisingly, the young heavy drinkers were more inclined than other teenagers to endorse 'positive' reasons for drinking. These included the belief that drinking facilitates talking to members of the opposite sex and mixing at parties. Heavy drinkers were also more likely than others to report drinking to calm their nerves and to relax or because of boredom. Heavy drinkers were more likely than others to report that all of their friends drank alcohol.

ADVERSE CONSEQUENCES

Several studies have obtained information about the possible consequences of youthful alcohol consumption. Jahoda and Cramond (1972) and Fossey (1992), as noted in Chapter 2, discovered that most young children are aware of drunkenness and that many form a rather hostile view of drinking. With the teenage years this is replaced, through peer pressure, personal experience and other factors, by a positive orientation towards alcohol.

Hawker (1978) reported that the majority of teenagers aged 13–18 in her survey had been intoxicated in the previous year. A minority reported experiencing hangover symptoms. Three per cent of the boys and 2 per cent of the girls reported having felt so ill during a hangover that they had missed a whole or half day at school or some other commitment. Seventeen per cent of the boys and 10 per cent of the girls reported having started a fight or argument after drinking heavily. Plant, Peck and Samuel (1985) examined the self-reported experiences of 15–16-year-olds in the Lothian Region. Seventy per cent of the boys and 61 per cent of the girls reported having at some time experienced a degree of intoxication. The general pattern of consequences reported by this study group is shown in Table 5.1.

As illustrated by this table, intoxication was commonplace and had, at least to a minor degree, been experienced by most of the teenagers who drank alcohol. A minority had also clearly experienced potentially serious consequences. These included arguments and accidents. Some had been advised by doctors to drink less and a small proportion had been worried about their drinking or had experienced what they regarded as problems.

The national survey by Marsh, Dobbs and White (1986) examined the extent of subjectively reported intoxication amongst teenagers. Even amongst the youngest age group surveyed, aged 13, the majority of both boys and girls reported having been 'a little bit drunk' at least once in the past year. Only amongst Scottish girls was such experience confined to a minority (46 per cent). By the age of 17 approximately 80 per cent of boys and the majority of girls (53–59 per cent) had been drunk at least once in the previous twelve months. Details were also elicited of the extent to which a variety of drink-related consequences had been experienced. The authors emphasized that most adolescents associated drinking with social enjoyment. They also concluded that adverse consequences were commonplace:

Table 5.1 Experience of some of the consequences of drinking amongst 15–16-year-olds in the Lothian Region (drinkers only)

Consequence	Males %	Females %
a) *Drunkenness*		
i) Have ever been 'merry', 'a little bit drunk' or 'very drunk'	70.4	61.0
ii) Having been 'merry' in past 6 weeks	62.9	57.8
iii) Having been 'a little bit drunk' in past 6 months	50.2	43.5
iv) Having been 'very drunk' in past 6 months	36.4	23.9
v) Have ever experienced hangover	30.6	26.3
vi) Having had hangover in past 6 months	25.5	22.6
vii) Had drunk in morning to steady nerves to get rid of hangover	5.5	3.0
b) *Health*		
i) Have been advised by doctor to drink less	2.1	1.3
ii) Have had alcohol-related accident/injury	8.9	5.1
iii) Have had 'upset stomach' due to drinking	40.2	28.9
iv) Have had shaky hand in morning after drinking	5.5	5.6
c) *Social*		
i) Have disagreed with parents because of drinking	18.5	20.1
ii) Have had own drinking criticized	17.2	11.2
iii) Have experienced school problems due to drinking	1.9	2.2
iv) Have spent too much on drink	26.4	14.2
v) Have quarrelled due to own drinking	11.3	8.4
vi) Have had financial problems due to own drinking	9.8	2.8
vii) Have arrived late at school due to drinking	2.3	2.2
d) *Self-ascription*		
i) Have been worried by own drinking	5.7	3.5
ii) Have experienced alcohol-related problems	7.9	4.4

Source: Plant *et al.* 1985: 30–1

Nearly half the 17 year old boys had been sick after drinking compared with 13% of the 17 year old girls. About a third of the oldest boys had also felt dizzy, confused, had a headache and 29% of the English and Welsh and 30% of the Scottish 17 year old boys managed to fall over, usually more than once. The corresponding figures for 17 year old girls are 11% and 7%.

(Marsh, Dobbs and White 1986: 43)

This study also indicated that younger adolescent girls were more likely to report adverse consequences than were older girls. Amongst the 14- and

15-year-olds, girls reported as many consequences as did the boys. The researchers examined the associations between the adverse and positive consequences of drinking, intoxication and drink-related problems. This analysis indicated that these were all associated. The researchers concluded:

> The incidence of positive experiences is quite closely related to that of negative experiences. The greater the degree of social enjoyment that adolescents recalled being associated with an evening's drinking, the more likely it was to have been followed by a disagreeable combination of sickness, incapacity and regret. Such symptoms, when they occurred often to adolescents, were closely associated with examples of anti-social behaviour when they too occurred.
>
> (Marsh, Dobbs and White 1986: 45)

It was concluded that teenagers are also able to drink and enjoy themselves without serious problems. Bagnall, referring to her survey of 13-year-olds, concluded that males reported: 'more frequent experience of the effects of alcohol, both positive and negative' (1988: 247).

OFFICIALLY RECORDED 'ALCOHOL PROBLEMS'

Some of the more conspicuous and serious adverse consequences of drinking are recorded by official agencies. It should be emphasized that very often the ill effects of excessive or inappropriate drinking are difficult to quantify. This is because the effects of the consumption of any drug, including alcohol, depend upon a complex interaction between the individual, the drug and the context (environment) in which use occurs. People react differently to drinking in different locations and individuals may vary greatly in their demeanour when under the influence of alcohol. It is often unclear, even if a person has been drinking heavily, to what extent a specific 'problem' or adverse consequence is due to drinking or to other factors. Researchers have, accordingly, often concluded that, although alcohol consumption is *associated* with crimes or other problems, it is difficult to prove a clear causal connection between drinking and its associated problems (e.g. Collins 1982).

Alcohol-related deaths

A comprehensive review of the role of alcohol in relation to mortality is beyond the scope of this book. Such reviews are available elsewhere (e.g. Royal College of Physicians 1987; Giesbrecht *et al.* 1989). 'Heavy drinking' is associated with a constellation of illnesses and deaths. For example, a considerable proportion of liver cirrhosis is associated with chronic heavy drinking. In addition, heavy drinking has also been associated with heart disease, cancers and other conditions. Apart from the toxic effects of prolonged high levels of alcohol, consumption of alcohol is also associated with accidents attributable to some extent to intoxication rather than to chronic alcohol consumption.

During 1988 three males and five females aged 24 or below died of chronic liver disease or cirrhosis in England and Wales. Two of these individuals, a male and a female, were below the age of one and so were not heavy drinkers. In Scotland during 1987 nobody under the age of 20 died from these conditions (Office of Population Censuses and Surveys 1990; Registrar General Scotland 1988).

The number of young people who die from *clearly* alcohol-related causes is relatively small. Here are some examples. During 1988 nobody under the age of 29 died from alcohol psychosis in England and Wales. However, two females and three males aged 15–24 died from the 'alcohol dependence syndrome'; three males and six females aged 15–24 died from the 'non-dependent abuse of alcohol'. One female aged between 20–24 died of alcoholic fatty liver. Nobody under the age of 24 died from acute alcoholic hepatitis or alcoholic cirrhosis of the liver. Three males and two females aged 15–24 died from the toxic effect of alcohol. Three males and two females aged 15–24 died from accidental poisoning by alcoholic beverage or by alcohol 'not elsewhere classified' (Office of Population Censuses and Surveys 1990; Registrar General Scotland 1988).

While few young people in Britain die from alcohol-related illnesses it is evident that larger numbers die in alcohol-related accidents. This is elaborated in the following section.

Alcohol and accidents

Alcohol, a depressant, is associated with accidents. This is, to a large extent, because the consumption of alcohol leads to the slowing of response times, combined with the mood changes associated with 'disinhibition'. The latter are discussed further in Chapter 10. A large number of studies have noted that alcohol consumption is associated with a significant proportion of accidents in the home, at work and in other contexts. The Royal College of Psychiatrists noted:

> In one study of 300 consecutive fatalities for unintentional injuries, however, 30 per cent of those dying were known to be heavy drinkers. A report from the Western Infirmary in Glasgow has shown that almost 50 per cent of the admissions for head injuries are the results of assaults

or falls while under the influence of alcohol and, at that hospital, admissions for such injuries are currently running at about 1,000 per year.

(Royal College of Psychiatrists 1986: 98–9)

The important, but complex, role of alcohol in relation to accidents and poisonings has recently been reviewed in detail by Giesbrecht *et al.* (1989).

Alcohol-related road accidents

Alcohol is implicated in a significant proportion of road traffic accidents (Ross 1982; Dunbar 1985; Havard 1986). Between 1979 and 1989 there was a marked *decline* in the proportion of younger people killed in British road accidents who were found to be over the legal blood alcohol limit for drivers (80 mg/100 ml). This is illustrated by Table 5.2.

As this table shows, the proportion of riders and drivers killed in the 16–19 age group with high blood alcohol levels fell by over 50 per cent between 1979–89. Moreover, in this group the highest proportion of people over the legal blood alcohol level were aged 20–39. As indicated by Table 5.2, during the decade following 1979 there had been a general fall in the proportion of deaths involving people with high blood alcohol levels. These fell from 31 per cent to 20 per cent amongst riders and from 32 per cent to

Table 5.2 Drivers and riders killed: percentages over the legal blood alcohol limit in Great Britain (1979–89)

Year	Two-wheeled motor vehicle riders Age groups				Drivers of cars and other motor vehicles Age groups			
	16–19 %	20–29 %	30–39 %	40+ %	16–19 %	20–29 %	30–39 %	40+ %
1979	26	40	46	19	34	42	47	20
1980	22	39	38	24	33	43	35	22
1981	16	39	38	29	20	45	39	20
1982	17	43	34	17	31	50	52	20
1983	17	29	30	8	34	42	43	14
1984	24	30	28	22	18	39	33	15
1985	15	27	39	11	25	40	38	14
1986	15	28	33	14	19	36	33	13
1987	16	31	24	16	16	32	27	13
1988	10	33	33	9	12	30	27	9
1989*	13	25	17	17	11	24	31	9

* Provisional figure
Source: Department of Transport 1990b: 25

19 per cent amongst drivers. It should be noted, however, that elevated blood alcohol levels are particularly high amongst pedestrians who are killed in road accidents. During 1988, 31 per cent of those aged 16–19 and 50 per cent of those aged 20–24 who were in this category were found to be over the legal blood alcohol level (Department of Transport 1990b).

During 1988, 946 people aged 19 or below died in road traffic accidents in England and Wales. In Scotland during 1987 the corresponding number was 114.

Alcohol and crime

The relationship between drinking and crime has been extensively considered and is complex. The general conclusion of available evidence is that alcohol use is *associated* with many crimes but that it is usually difficult to identify a clear causal relationship. Neither feelings nor behaviours are found in a bottle. Drinking does not by itself produce criminal behaviour. The effects of alcohol, or any psychoactive drug, are influenced by a variety of factors. These include the chemistry of the substance or substances used, the characteristics of the user and the context in which use occurs (e.g. Collins 1982; Myers 1983, 1986).

Alcohol is a depressant drug. One of the characteristic features of consuming alcohol is that it may lead to 'disinhibition'. This has been defined as the 'activation of behaviours normally suppressed by various controlling influences' (Woods and Mansfield 1983: 4).

Room has described the popular view of alcohol-induced disinhibition thus:

It is commonplace in our culture that alcohol is a disinhibitor – that drunkenness not only makes one clumsy, but also removes social constraints, makes us, for instance, aggressive or affectionate, maudlin or mean, in a way we would not be if we were sober. Often a pseudo-scientific explanation is given: 'Alcohol depresses the higher centers of the brain'. Such 'explanations' reflect the wide and popular and professional belief that disinhibition is a pharmacological property of alcohol. In everyday language and life, this presumed pharmacological action is often used to excuse or account for otherwise inexcusable behaviour.

(Room 1983: v)

Youthful drinking, as indicated above, not infrequently leads to intoxication. As shown, for example, by Table 5.1, a minority of adolescents report having at some time been involved with arguments which they attribute to their own drinking. Myers (1982) has concluded that alcohol use is a frequent precursor to or accompaniment of violent acts. In addition,

Myers noted that it is often the victim as well as the assailant who has been drinking at the time of an assault.

Young men, drunk or sober, form a large proportion of those who are convicted of crimes and in particular crimes of violence. Periodically, public disorder involving young people has been linked with alcohol or illicit drugs. During 1987 and 1988 politicians and the police voiced concern about public disorder in a number of small towns in England and Wales. It was noted that such disorder frequently involved young people who were drunk. This problem led to the conduct of a study to investigate these disorderly episodes. The resulting report (Tuck 1989) examined violent outbreaks which had occurred over a wide geographical area. Three 'trouble sites' were compared with locations where no trouble had been reported. It was concluded that disorder was more likely to occur outside licensed premises after drinking rather than in such premises:

> Young people leave pubs en masse at the same hour, emerge on to the streets still looking for further entertainment, cluster at fast-food outlets or at other gathering points and are at this point excitable tinder, ready for any spark which may cause quarrels or violence.
>
> (Tuck 1989: 66)

Tuck noted that, though weekend drinking was a routine social habit amongst young people, only a minority became involved in violence:

> Participants in disorder are more likely to have unskilled jobs or to be unemployed. . . . and to have left school at sixteen. These are young men who have not yet found their role in society. They may not have enough money to go on to night-clubs after their evening in the pub (even if they exist in their vicinity); they cluster outside take-aways, unwilling for the evening to end, still looking for excitement. It is these gatherings which are the characteristic focus of disorder.
>
> (Tuck 1989: 66)

Tuck suggested that the managers of licensed premises and fast-food chains and planning authorities could usefully seek to reduce 'congestion sites'. She also concluded that:

> the 'disco pub' or 'youth pub' may be a particular source of excitement and that perhaps consideration should be given to changing the rules under which these establishments operate. At present they are far less controlled than establishments with late night music and dancing licences.
>
> (Tuck 1989: 67)

Tuck also noted that most, but not all, of the disorderly incidents examined were linked to alcohol use by young people.

In 1989 in England and Wales 92,822 people were cautioned for, or were found guilty of, drunkenness offences. In 1981 the corresponding figure had been higher, 97,890. Approximately 6 per cent of those cautioned or convicted in 1989 were aged 17 or below and 15 per cent were aged 18–20 years.

In 1989, the peak age of offending for drunkenness offences was 20 years for males and females. The rate of offending was 1,140 per 100,000 population for males and 77 per 100,000 for females. The rate of offending for those aged under 18, the minimum legal age for consumption of alcohol in a bar or licensed premises and for the purchase of alcohol from off-licences, was 140 per 100,000 population.

(Home Office 1990a: 2)

Over 70 per cent of those cautioned for or found guilty of drunkenness offences were in the major metropolitan counties. It was noted that there has recently been an increase in the use of cautioning (rather than conviction) for drunkenness offences. Relatively few convictions in England and Wales relate to those offences specifically concerned with 'under age drinking':

The number of persons convicted under section 169 (2) (persons under 18 buying intoxicating liquor) fell by 40 per cent to 520 in 1989 following a sharp rise from 540 in 1987 to 900 in 1988. A total of 2,310 persons were either found guilty or cautioned for this offence, similar to that in 1986, the latest year for which comparable data is available. The number of licensees convicted under section 169 (1) of selling intoxicating liquor to persons under 18 rose by 9 per cent from 360 in 1988 to 390 in 1989.

(Home Office 1990a: 4)

The number of young people in England and Wales who were found guilty of drunkenness offences between 1981 and 1989 is shown in Table 5.3.

As this table shows, the numbers of young females found guilty of drunkenness offences in England and Wales remained fairly stable between 1981 and 1986. The number of males found guilty of such offences also remained little changed until 1986. In 1986 numbers fell to 39,613. During 1987, 1988 and 1989 there was an increase in the number of males and females ages 21–30 who were found guilty. This figure is at least partly attributable to the introduction of the Sporting Events (Control of Alcohol etc. . .) Act. This came into effect in July 1985 and introduced the new offences of being drunk on a vehicle or when entering a designated sporting event. Such changes in legislation can exert a considerable effect on levels of officially recorded crimes. The Criminal Justice (Scotland) Act (1980)

Table 5.3 Young people in England and Wales found guilty or cautioned for offences of drunkenness (1981–89)

Sex and age	1981	1982	1983	1984	1985	1986	1987	1988	1989
Males									
Under 18	4,425	4,541	4,796	4,759	4,607	4,020	4,427	4,254	3,357
18 and under 21	15,083	14,961	15,183	13,971	14,143	12,450	14,658	15,037	13,425
21 and under 30	22,083	21,764	22,611	20,363	20,412	19,143	24,911	29,412	29,188
Total	41,591	41,266	42,590	39,093	39,162	35,613	43,996	48,703	45,970
Females									
Under 18	429	453	419	433	457	438	439	436	416
18 and under 21	920	799	800	766	744	665	812	852	842
21 and under 30	2,001	1,811	1,798	1,604	1,381	1,269	1,708	1,876	1,960
Total	3,350	3,063	3,017	2,803	2,582	2,372	2,959	3,164	3,218

Source: Home Office 1990a: 8

restricted the carriage, sale and consumption of alcohol at sporting events, in particular football matches, and on public transport associated with sport. This legislation also extended the decriminalization of public drunkenness in Scotland. Since the introduction of the new law some people who would formerly have been convicted of public order offences have been referred to facilities such as detoxification centres.

In conclusion, alcohol misuse amongst young people has become established as a chronic problem in the United Kingdom. During the past decade both the use and misuse of alcohol by young people have stabilized and there is some evidence of a *decline* in the levels of alcohol-related problems, such as those related to drunken driving. It is emphasized that the great majority of young people in Britain do consume alcohol and that most during their teenage years experience intoxication and other mild adverse consequences associated with drinking. Recent surveys suggest that a minority of teenagers do drink relatively heavily and that those individuals are especially 'at risk' in relation to adverse consequences. Alcohol misuse is associated with a substantial proportion of accidents, deaths and public order offences, though the precise role of alcohol in relation to such problems is often unclear. The overwhelming majority of alcohol-related problems amongst young people relate neither to chronic heavy drinking nor to alcohol dependence but to the ill effects of acute intoxication.

6 Tobacco-related harm

Tobacco smoking is responsible for more adverse health effects than any other psychoactive drug. The scale of tobacco-related ill health is massive. Strangely, it was not until the 1950s that clear and persuasive evidence of the adverse effects of tobacco was produced. This related to the association between tobacco smoking and lung cancer, heart disease, emphysema and chronic bronchitis (Doll and Hill 1952, 1964; World Health Organization 1960; Anderson and Ferris 1962; Wynder and Hoffman 1967; Doll and Peto 1986).

The health toll inflicted by tobacco use has been indicated by the Royal College of Physicians:

At present tobacco still accounts for 15 to 20 per cent of all British deaths. Precise calculation is not easy, but with reasonable assumptions the annual death toll in the United Kingdom will not be less than 100,000. This figure is so large that it completely dwarfs the number of deaths that can be reliably attributed to any other known external factors such as alcohol, road accidents, suicide etc. . . . Appreciation of the magnitude of the problem is helped by putting the figures in the context of hazards that people already have some feelings for, thus: Among 1,000 young adult males in England and Wales who smoke cigarettes on average about

1 will be murdered
6 will be killed on the roads
250 will be killed before their time by tobacco.
(Royal College of Physicians 1986: 2)

The Royal College of Physicians also noted:

Besides death must be set the misery to its victims of prolonged ill health, loss of working time and cost to the nation. Sickness due to cigarette smoking leads to the loss of an estimated 50 million working days each year, about four times that due to strikes.

(Royal College of Physicians 1986: 2)

Tobacco smoking has been implicated in approximately a third of British cancer deaths and 90 per cent of lung cancer deaths. Tobacco is a highly dependence (or 'addiction') producing drug. Russell (1974) declared that it is probably the most addictive of all known drugs. This view has recently been questioned by Henningfield, Cohen and Slade (1991). Even so, these researchers, comparing nicotine and cocaine, reached the conclusion that, though nicotine did not appear to be 'more addictive' than cocaine:

Both are highly addicting drugs for which patterns of use and the development of dependence are strongly influenced by factors such as availability, price, social pressures, and regulations, as well as certain pharmacologic characteristics.

(Henningfield, Cohen and Slade 1991: 565)

The United States Surgeon General (1988) produced a report which stated that tobacco was as 'addictive' as heroin or cocaine. This document has recently been reviewed by West and Grunberg (1991). These authors noted that, while in some respects tobacco research has made advances, tobacco use is continuing to *increase* worldwide:

as a prerequisite for making substantial inroads into tobacco related disease, governments need to be persuaded to take the problem seriously and to take action which is within their power to reduce tobacco use prevalence.

(West and Grunberg 1991: 488)

Some of the recent British evidence on trends in youthful tobacco use has been briefly reviewed in Chapter 3. As indicated therein tobacco use has been declining. In spite of this approximately a third of the adult British population still smoke and over a quarter of those aged 16–19 do so.

The decline in tobacco use in the United Kingdom has been reflected by a clear reduction in tobacco-related ill health. Frogatt has also noted that the lower tar content of modern cigarettes has led to 'reductions in the risk of lung cancer from 40 to 20%' (1988: 17). This fall has been docu- mented in detail by Wald, Doll and Copeland (1981) and by Wald and Frogatt (1988). Frogatt (1988) has elaborated the scale of the difference in risk associated with different tar levels in cigarettes:

Secular trends in lung cancer in England and Wales confirm that the risk of lung cancer is reduced in smokers of lower tar cigarettes. This is seen most clearly among the younger age groups, whose smoking histories will have been less dominated by the higher yielding products of earlier decades. Among men aged 30–34 lung cancer mortality during 1980–84 was only a third of that in 1950–54. Over the same interval the consumption of cigarettes in that group fell to two-thirds of its former value, while tar yields fell to about half of the levels that prevailed up to the early 1950s.

(Frogatt 1988: 16)

In spite of these obvious improvements tobacco use continues to inflict enormous health damage. During 1988 over 70,000 people in England and Wales died of cancers of the bronchus, trachea or lung. In the same year over 4,000 people in Scotland died from the same causes. During 1988 over 30,000 people in Scotland and over 249,000 people in England and Wales died from ischaemic heart disease or from acute myocardial infarction. A high proportion of those deaths were tobacco-related. Fewer than 100 of the deaths involved people aged 29 or younger. Even so there is no doubt that many tobacco-related deaths are attributable to the adoption of cigarette smoking while at an early age (Office of Population Censuses and Surveys 1990; Registrar General Scotland 1989). The great majority of those who die from cancers of the bronchus, trachea or lung are middle-aged or elderly. Even so, a minority are in their twenties or thirties or even younger. During 1988, 246 people aged 39 or younger died from these conditions in England and Wales.

PASSIVE SMOKING

There is no doubt that tobacco smoking is harmful to the smoker. Evidence also indicates that maternal smoking during pregnancy has adverse effects on foetal development. This is elaborated in Chapter 8. It is now apparent that 'passive' or 'involuntary' smoking also has harmful effects. This involves non-smokers being exposed to the smoke from cigarettes or other tobacco products smoked by other people. In 1987 the Independent Scientific Committee on Smoking and Health produced a statement to the effect that passive smoking was associated with a small increase in lung cancer risk.

Frogatt (1988) has reviewed recent evidence on passive smoking or 'environmental tobacco smoke'. He concluded that most studies indicated that passive smoking is associated with an increase in the risk of lung cancer. Even so, a minority of investigations have concluded that such effects are negligible or even non-existent. Frogatt and his Committee agreed with the view that passive smoking does raise many cancer risks in the range of 10–30 per cent.

ARE YOUNG PEOPLE HARMED BY TOBACCO?

Most, but not all, of those who die from tobacco-related diseases are middle-aged and elderly. It is emphasized that, although some young people do die from such causes, tobacco-related premature death is usually a long-term consequence of a continued smoking career. Tobacco smoking causes widespread ill health in addition to its fatal effects. Smoking is associated not only with cancers, but with heart disease, bronchitis and a number of other ailments. Even young children who smoke report higher levels of respiratory symptoms than do non-smokers (Bewley and Bland 1976; Bland *et al.* 1978). Children who smoke often have coughs which most recognize as being associated with their smoking. Young heavier smokers also report more frequent coughs, colds and shortness of breath than do non-smokers (Bewley and Bland 1978; Seely, Zuskin and Bonhuys 1971). Teenage smokers also have reduced lung function and other respiratory abnormalities (Seely, Zuskin and Bonhuys 1971; Niewoehner, Kleinerman and Rice 1974). The Royal College of Physicians (1986) has noted that children are harmed not only by their own smoking, but also by that of their parents. This is reflected in increased rates of pneumonia and bronchitis:

> There is a clear link between the number of cigarettes smoked by parents and the frequency of such illness, which cannot be explained in terms of perinatal illness, breast feeding or poor housing and social conditions.
>
> (Royal College of Physicians 1986: 57)

Rona, Chin and Du V Florey (1985) distinguished between the effects on children of maternal smoking during pregnancy and subsequent exposure to parental smoking. They concluded that parental smoking was associated with decreased child height. This analysis controlled for social class and a number of other factors.

It has been noted in Chapter 3 that young people in the lowest socio-economic groups are those most likely to smoke. This connection between smoking and socio-economic status persists in the later stages of life. Both short-term respiratory symptoms, absence from school or work and longer-term, increasingly serious illnesses as well as premature deaths are clearly and directly attributable to tobacco use. Although smoking is not exclusively confined to those in lower socio-economic groups it imposes a disproportionate toll on those who have low incomes and who are often otherwise seriously disadvantaged in a variety of ways. Young people who are smokers are also more likely to use illicit drugs and to drink heavily. Young people from lower socio-economic backgrounds, as emphasized by Jessor and Jessor (1977), are 'at risk' in relation to a number of problem behaviours. These connections are discussed further in Chapter 11.

To reiterate, tobacco continues to be associated with massive health damage. The scale of this dwarfs the health effects associated with alcohol or illicit drugs. Most of the serious consequences of tobacco smoking do not become apparent until the middle and later years of life. Even so some health damage, such as bronchitis, is evident amongst young smokers. In addition, 'passive smoking' involves harm to people who do not smoke and, as elaborated in Chapter 8, maternal smoking in pregnancy is also harmful.

It is certainly a problem that the ill effects of tobacco are often not evident in the short term. This fact is probably a barrier, or at least an impediment, to health education and to the desired objective of discouraging people from smoking. In spite of this, as indicated by Chapter 3, there has been a dramatic and steady fall in smoking in Britain during recent years. Even now over a quarter of the adult population continue to indulge in this especially dangerous behaviour.

7   Drug-related harm

This chapter relates to illicit drugs such as cannabis, LSD, heroin and cocaine as well as substances such as glues and solvents. As noted in Chapter 4, the latter are not 'illegal' in the same sense as substances covered by the Misuse of Drugs Act (1971). It is difficult, as outlined in the two preceding chapters, to measure the extent of the adverse consequences of legal drug use. It is even harder to measure the adverse consequences of using illicit drugs, the very use of which is only partly evident. Accordingly, only a partial picture is available. As already noted, though many young people do at sometime use illicit drugs, most do so only on a strictly temporary and limited basis. Regular or 'heavy' use is restricted to a small minority. It is therefore not surprising that most of those who use illicit drugs do not come to the attentions of 'official agencies' because of their use of these substances. Those who do come to such attention are particularly likely to be those who use drugs most often.

Two key indicators of drug misuse are available. The first of these relates to 'addicts' notified to the Home Office and the second to cautions and convictions for drug offences. Both of these indicators provide a useful measure of specific trends over time. Even so, the limitations of these statistics have recently been emphasized by the Home Office:

> The number of addicts who are notified to the Home Office is probably only a small proportion of the number of regular misusers. Many will not have sought medical treatment and will not therefore have been notified. Researchers have demonstrated that there are considerable local variations in the extent to which the number of notified addicts under-estimate the number of regular users of notifiable drugs. It may also be that for a variety of reasons, doctors do not notify all the addicts that they see.
>
> (Home Office 1990b: 1)

Comparable limitations apply to official records of people cautioned or convicted of drug offences. These are certainly influenced by a variety of factors, such as local variations in police policy and alternative demands upon police resources.

ADDICT NOTIFICATIONS

As outlined in Chapter 4, during the early decades of the twentieth century very few people were officially recorded as dependent upon morphine, heroin and allied drugs. This situation changed during the 1960s. During the past two decades there has been a marked increase in the number of recorded addicts. This is shown in Table 7.1.

As this table indicates, addict notifications have risen more than tenfold since 1970. The rate of increase has varied, but in many years between 1970 and 1989 it exceeded 10 per cent. It exceeded 20 per cent in two years. The

Table 7.1 Narcotic addicts known to the Home Office (1970–90)*

Year	Males	Females	Total	Change over previous years
1970	1,051	375	1,426	–
1971	1,133	416	1,549	+ 9%
1972	1,195	421	1,616	+ 4%
1973	1,370	446	1,816	+12%
1974	1,458	509	1,967	+ 8%
1975	1,438	511	1,949	– 1%
1976	1,387	487	1,874	– 4%
1977	1,466	550	2,016	+ 8%
1978	1,703	699	2,402	+19%
1979	1,892	774	2,666	+11%
1980	2,009	837	2,846	+ 7%
1981	2,732	1,112	3,844	+35%
1982	3,124	1,247	4,371	+14%
1983	3,601	1,478	5,079	+16%
1984	4,133	1,736	5,869	+15%
1985	4,952	2,100	7,052	+20%
1986	5,325	2,810	8,135	+15%
1987	7,766	2,950	10,716	+31%
1988	9,093	3,551	12,644	+18%
1989	10,479	4,306	14,789	+17%
1990	12,807	4,948	17,755	+20%

* At 31 December each year
Figures are rounded to nearest %
Source: Home Office 1979–91

proportion of notified addicts who were female remained relatively stable throughout this period, at just over a quarter.

Most notified addicts are young. As indicated by Table 7.2, during 1989 the average age of female addicts was 28.3 and that of males was 29.2.

During 1989, 67 per cent of addicts from whom relevant data were elicited were classified as injectors and 33 per cent were classified as non-injectors. Males were marginally more likely than females to be recorded as injectors, 69 per cent compared with 62 per cent.

Home Office statistics revealed that marked variations existed in the rates of addict notifications in relation to overall population. These were particularly high in London, Merseyside, Greater Manchester, Cheshire, Lancashire, Norfolk and the Lothian and Borders regions in Scotland.

Most notified addicts are recorded as being dependent upon heroin or methadone. This is elaborated in Table 7.3.

During the past two decades there has been a steady increase in the number of people recorded in each year who are 'new addicts'. These increased from 9 per cent between 1970–8 to 37 per cent in 1988. The highest rates of new heroin addicts recorded in 1989 were in London, Merseyside and Greater Manchester.

DRUG OFFENCES

During 1945 the Home Office recorded 200 offences related to opium, four related to cannabis and twenty for manufactured drugs. In 1989, 38,415 persons were found guilty, cautioned or dealt with by compounding for

Table 7.2 Age distribution of narcotic drug addicts notified to the Home Office in 1989

Age	Males	Females
Under 21	954	489
21 and under 25	2,310	1,070
25 and under 30	3,058	1,274
30 and under 35	1,965	789
35 and under 50	1,987	594
50 and over	93	50
Not recorded	112	40
Total all ages	10,479	4,306
Average age	29.2	28.3

Source: Home Office 1990b

Table 7.3 Type of drug to which addiction was notified in 1989

Drug	Number of persons
Heroin	12,484
Methadone	2,951
Dipipanone (Diconal)	349
Cocaine	888
Morphine	760
Pethidine	85
Dextromoramide	266
Levorphanol	1
Oxycodone	2
Phenazocine	5
Opium	25

Note An individual can be notified as addicted to more than one drug. These figures cannot be added to produce the total number of people recorded.
Source: Home Office 1990b

drug offences in the United Kingdom. Table 7.4 provides details of the marked increase in such offences that occurred between 1979 and 1989.

As this table shows, the great majority of drug offenders are charged in relation to cannabis offences. During 1989 the latter accounted for 87.6 per cent of individual cases. Heroin was involved in far fewer cases, fewer than 5 per cent.

Most drug offenders are young. Between 1979 and 1989 their average age in any year ranged from 25.2 to 25.9. Most drug offenders are also male. In 1989 only 10.2 per cent were female. The age distribution of drug offenders during 1989 is shown in Table 7.5.

DRUG-RELATED MORTALITY

A review by Ghodse *et al.* (1985) concluded that between 1967 and 1981, 1,499 'notified addicts' in the United Kingdom had died. This mortality was sixteen times greater than that expected for people of comparable age. Other authors have reported that institutionalized 'problem drug users' have a mortality ranging from 1–2 per cent per year (e.g. Thorley 1981; Stimson and Oppenheimer 1982; Bucknall and Robertson 1986). Other researchers have reported higher mortality rates (e.g. Jamieson, Glanz and MacGregor 1984).

During 1988 sixty-nine males and sixteen females aged 24 or less died from 'drug dependence' in England and Wales. In addition, thirteen males

Table 7.4 Persons* found guilty, cautioned or dealt with by compounding for drugs offences by drug type

Type of drug	1979	1980	1981	1982	1983	1984	1985	1986	1987	1988	1989
Cocaine	331	476	566	426	563	698	632	449	518	591	786
Dipipanone	453	440	498	566	370	252	97	59	70	44	44
Heroin	520	751	808	966	1,508	2,446	3,227	2,259	2,151	1,856	1,769
LSD	208	246	345	466	451	558	539	286	300	240	435
Methadone	299	363	445	404	379	411	413	280	191	162	172
Amphetamines	760	827	1,074	1,521	2,008	2,501	2,946	2,655	2,299	2,538	2,395
Cannabis	12,409	14,912	15,388	17,447	20,066	20,746	21,337	19,286	21,733	26,111	33,669
Other	1,163	1,288	1,141	1,008	947	976	1,023	952	1,167	1,222	1,263
All drugs	14,339	17,158	17,921	20,356	23,442	25,240	26,958	23,905	26,278	30,515	38,415

* As the same person may be found guilty, cautioned or dealt with by compounding for offences involving more than one drug, columns cannot be added together to produce sub-totals or totals.
Source : Home Office 1990c

Table 7.5 Age distribution of persons found guilty, cautioned or dealt with by compounding for drugs offences

Age	Males	Females
Under 17	1,171	141
17 and under 21	9,580	898
21 and under 25	9,538	1,026
25 and under 30	7,225	884
30 and over	6,968	984
Total	34,482	3,933

Source: Home Office 1990c

and three females in this age group died from the 'non-dependent abuse of drugs'. In the same year twenty-two males and six females aged 24 or less died from poisoning by opiates and related narcotics, barbiturates and benzodiazepine-based tranquillizers (Office of Population Censuses and Surveys 1990). In Scotland four males aged 24 or less died of 'drug dependence' in 1988. A further two males in this age group died from the non-dependent abuse of drugs. Three males and one female died from 'accidental poisoning by drugs, medicaments and biologicals'. It was also concluded that four Scottish deaths had resulted from 'solvent abuse'. Accidental deaths involving heroin, morphine and methadone were noted in eight cases. Suicidal (i.e. intentional) deaths frequently involved drugs, often in combination with alcohol. It is also possible that other deaths may be drug-related. These, such as road traffic accidents, often involve a variety of causal factors (Registrar General Scotland 1989).

The Home Office has provided details of recent deaths related to drug misuse:

In 1989 there were 1,200 deaths in the United Kingdom where the underlying cause was attributed to drug dependence or non-dependent abuse of drugs or controlled drugs were somehow implicated as a cause. Some 250 deaths were attributed to drug dependence or non-dependent abuse of drugs (other than alcohol or tobacco). A further 200 deaths resulted from accidental poisoning by controlled drugs and 280 involved poisoning by controlled drugs with 'undetermined external cause'. In addition some 430 people committed suicide with the aid of controlled drugs. The number of deaths from AIDS where the person was known to be an injecting drug user at 18 was small but twice the number in 1987.

Injecting drug users are now one of the more rapidly increasing exposure categories among cases of AIDS.

(Home Office 1991: 11–12)

The annual number of deaths amongst 'notified addicts' rose from 124 in 1979 to 296 in 1989. During the latter year the pattern of deaths was as shown in Table 7.6. At least three Ecstasy-related deaths were noted in 1991.

HIV INFECTION AND AIDS

The mortality associated with illicit drug use has been transformed by the advent of AIDS. As noted elsewhere in this book, one of the major methods whereby HIV infection is transmitted is the sharing of infected injecting equipment by drug users (e.g. Strang and Stimson 1990). In some localities, such as Edinburgh, the majority of cases of detected HIV infection and AIDS are attributable to injected drug use.

Intravenous drug users constituted 32 per cent of AIDS cases reported from thirty-two European countries up to 23 May 1990 (Brenner, Hernando-Briongos and Goos 1991). These authors noted that HIV sero-prevalence amongst intravenous drug users ranged from 0.0007 per cent in the USSR to 30–80 per cent in Italy, 40–69 per cent in Spain, 15–37 per cent in Switzerland, 30 per cent in Amsterdam and up to 30–60 per cent in the United Kingdom.

Table 7.6 Deaths of UK drug addicts in 1989*

Cause of Death	Number
Not primarily associated with drug misuse (n = 114)	
Natural	49
Accident	36
Homicide victim	1
Suicide	17
Not known	11
Associated with drug misuse (n = 182)	
Overdose	148
Other drug-related	26
HIV/AIDS	8
Total	296

* This table relates only to individuals notified to the Home Office. Other data indicate that eighteen UK AIDS deaths during 1989 involved intravenous drug users.
Source: Home Office 1991

At the end of 1990, 945 out of 1,840 people in Scotland who were recorded as HIV infected were intravenous drug users. Over 60 per cent of these HIV seropositive drug users were recorded in Edinburgh (*n*=578), Dundee (*n*=182) and Glasgow (*n*=153). Sixty-eight per cent of the Scottish HIV infected drug users were in the age range 20–29. Between 1984 and the end of 1990, 2,017 out of 15,166 cases of HIV infection in the United Kingdom were attributed solely to intravenous drug use (Answer 1991a, 1991b). The AIDS epidemic is still in its infancy. Even so, an alarming picture is already developing:

> For the population as a whole, AIDS deaths in England and Wales for 1989 were approximately one tenth of those for road traffic accidents and one fifth of those for all infectious and parasitic diseases combined . . . . The Scottish rates for 1989 were approximately one half of those for England and Wales.

> (Answer 1991b: 1)

During January 1991 the World Health Organization reported that 323,378 AIDS cases had been recorded of which 45,737 were from Europe (Answer 1991b: 4). By September 1990 a total of 2,040 AIDS deaths had been recorded in the United Kingdom. Fifty-eight of these, 3 per cent, were recorded as intravenous drug users. In addition, thirty individuals, 1 per cent, were recorded as intravenous drug users who were also bisexual or homosexual males. In addition, intravenous drug use was noted in relation to 15 per cent of a total of 117 HIV-infected people who had died but who did not have AIDS (Answer 1990b).

Intravenous drug use plays a bigger role in relation to HIV infection and AIDS in Scotland than in other areas of the United Kingdom. By 31 December 1989 intravenous drug users accounted for only 1.7 per cent of AIDS cases in England, Wales and Northern Ireland. The Scottish proportion was 25.7 per cent (Answer 1990a).

Between 1985 and 1989 the annual number of AIDS-related deaths amongst intravenous drug users in the United Kingdom rose from one case to eighteen. During the same period the total annual number of AIDS deaths in the UK rose from 119 to 567 (Home Office 1991).

As noted elsewhere in this book, those who use illicit drugs heavily are often also heavy users of alcohol, tobacco and prescribed drugs. Some individuals experience adverse consequences from drug use but do not seek agency help. In addition, some illicit drug users also experience severe alcohol-related problems (Morrison and Plant 1990, 1991). People from lower socio-economic backgrounds generally use health care facilities less than those from higher socio-economic backgrounds. This certainly biases the types of records kept by 'official agencies'.

To conclude, it appears that during recent decades there has been a steady and considerable increase in both the use and misuse of illicit drugs. This has been accompanied by an increase in levels of drug-related harm, including premature death amongst young drug misusers. Because illicit drugs are far less widely used than alcohol or tobacco the problems associated with such substances involve far fewer people. Even so, as noted above, over 1,200 deaths per year have recently been linked with illicit drugs. The potential health risks associated with illicit drugs have been hugely magnified by the spread of HIV infection through the sharing of infected injecting equipment. In some British cities, and elsewhere, this has been the fastest spreading mode of HIV infection. This targets not only intravenous drug users, but also their unborn children, their sexual partners and thereby the entire community.

8 Alcohol, drugs and pregnancy

The possibility that alcohol might be injurious if consumed during pregnancy has been acknowledged for centuries. The Bible and the Talmud advised pregnant women to refrain from drinking. In the ancient city states of Sparta and Carthage alcohol consumption was proscribed for all males and females 30 or younger who were recently married. This rule was intended to prevent the conception of damaged children (Haggard and Jellinek 1942; Plant 1985). It is clear that the development of the human foetus may be adversely effected, even terminated, by exposure to a wide range of chemical compounds (Elkington 1986).

Sometimes, as noted elsewhere in this book, people use several types of drug in combination. During the eighteenth century opium use was both legal and widespread in Britain. The offspring of opium-using mothers were described as 'poor wizened, ill-nourished' and 'pitiable to behold' (Berridge and Edwards 1981). The babies of mothers who drank heavily were described in very similar terms: 'starved, shrivel'd and imperfect as though . . . numbered many years' (Coffey 1966). Polydrug use or multiple drug use is discussed elsewhere in this book. This phenomenon greatly confuses the task of determining the effect of any specific psychoactive drug.

The use of alcohol during pregnancy was once fostered, not only by the usual social pressures to drink, but to improve maternal nutrition. Alcohol was recognized as a possible risk factor during pregnancy but was also accepted as treatment for premature labour. It was used as a painkiller during childbirth (Warner and Rosett 1975) and recommended as an aid to women wishing to breastfeed, the notion being that alcohol helps the 'let down reflex' whereby the milk becomes available to the baby. In fact, the opposite is the case as alcohol inhibits this process.

One of the first serious investigations of the possible influence of drinking during pregnancy was conducted by Sullivan in Liverpool, England. This study examined females in a Liverpool prison. The investigator concluded that 'the death rate amongst the children of inebriate mothers was nearly two and a half times that amongst the infants of sober women of the same stock' (Sullivan 1899).

Interest in the possible link between maternal drinking and foetal harm waned during the early part of the twentieth century, presumably reflecting the falling alcohol consumption associated with the First World War and the Depression of the 1930s. Haggard and Jellinek (1942) referred to this topic, but concluded that available evidence failed to provide tangible evidence. Their view was reaffirmed by Montague (1965) who stated that, on the basis of 'hundreds of studies covering many years', alcohol consumed by either father or mother did not appear to affect the development of the human foetus. However, where Montague's 'hundreds of studies' were carried out remains a mystery. In spite of this firm conclusion, the topic of drinking during pregnancy continued to stimulate scientific interest. Several studies were published in the 1950s and 1960s (e.g. Roquette 1957; Christiaens, Mizon and Demarle 1960; Christiaens 1961). A French study was described by Lemoine *et al.* (1968). This investigation, which related to 127 children of mothers or fathers who were problem drinkers, was important. The authors failed to differentiate between maternal and paternal alcohol problems. Even so, they described a syndrome of clinical features associated with the offspring of alcohol-dependent people. These included low birth weight and intelligence, short height, slow growth, language and psychomotor delays. The authors also noted that these children had a characteristic facial appearance. They were distinguished by a sunken nasal bridge, short upturned nose and malformed ears. Ulleland *et al.* (1970) and Ulleland (1972) reported a failure to thrive amongst a small study group of sixteen children of alcohol-abusing mothers in the USA.

Jones and Smith (1973), working with Ulleland, suggested a name for the features associated with the characteristics of the offspring of alcohol dependent mothers, the *Fetal Alcohol Syndrome*. These authors, echoing the earlier work of Lemoine *et al.* (1968), listed the characteristics associated with this syndrome. These included pre- and postnatal growth deficiency, short palpebral fissure size and developmental delays. Other common traits included joint and heart abnormalities, microcephaly and fine motor dysfunction. Distinctive facial features were again noted. These included receding forehead and chin, upturned nose and asymmetrical ears. This appearance is illustrated by Figure 8.1.

This paper, introducing in formal terms a new syndrome, was a very influential publication. It exerted an impact which, unlike earlier reports, was world-wide. It should be emphasized that Jones and Smith (1973) based their report on only eleven cases which had been examined in Seattle by Ulleland. Moreover, the precise aetiology of the babies' appearances

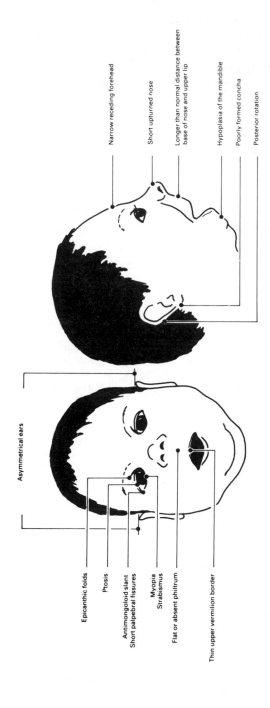

Figure 8.1 Features of the Fetal Alcohol Syndrome

Source: Plant (1985)

and characteristics was debatable. To determine what causes such a 'syndrome' it is necessary to examine many possible factors which were simply beyond the scope of the initial study. It is risky to name a syndrome after what may (or may not) cause it. The mothers of the first eight of these eleven children had been diagnosed as 'alcoholic' with problem drinking careers ranging from two to twenty-three years. Five of these had experienced delirium tremens (two during pregnancy) and one of the children had been born 'while her mother was in an alcoholic stupor' (Jones *et al.* 1973). The authors emphasized that these children had mothers who were extreme and atypical in relation to their drinking habits. In spite of this fact, alarm about the possible effects of alcohol use during pregnancy spread to include all levels and patterns of alcohol consumption. Eight years later, before the results of any large-scale studies had been published, the United States Surgeon General issued the following statement:

> Even if she does not bear a child with the full Fetal Alcohol Syndrome (FAS) a women who drinks heavily is more likely to bear a child with one or more of the birth defects included in the Syndrome. . . . Each patient should be told about the risk of alcohol consumption during pregnancy and advised not to drink alcoholic beverages and to be aware of the alcoholic content of food and drugs.
>
> (United States Surgeon General 1981: 9–40)

This advice – for all pregnant women to refrain from drinking – was from the outset controversial. The work of Lemoine *et al.* and Jones and Smith and their co-workers stimulated a considerable number of studies in many countries. These generally confirmed both the existence, and the rarity, of the Fetal Alcohol Syndrome (e.g. Hayder and Nelson 1978; Dehaene *et al.* 1977; Olegard *et al.* 1979; Mena *et al.* 1980; Majewski 1981; Halliday, Reid and McClure 1982; Poskitt, Hensey and Smith 1982; Beattie *et al.* 1983). Most of these studies tried to assess the frequency of its occurrence but did not address to the issue of what might cause the syndrome. In order to examine this several large-scale prospective studies have been conducted.

The US National Institute for Alcohol Abuse and Alcoholism (NIAAA) has funded four major studies which have been described elsewhere (e.g. Streissguth *et al.* 1987). These, together with other studies, have produced an extensive array of data, largely elicited from women attending antenatal clinics. Unlike much of the initial work on this topic, several investigations have attempted to examine and to control for the possible effects of tobacco and illicit drug use, together with other 'confounding' factors such as socio-economic status, diet, age and health. Some investigations have also addressed the issue of whether or not birth defects are associated with specific types of alcoholic beverage. Kuzma and Sokol (1982) concluded that heavy beer consumption by pregnant women was associated with decreased intrauterine growth. Wine consumption related only to decreased birth weight. A major study in Boston has been described by Rosett, Weiner and Edelin (1983). The majority of the subjects in this study were poor, black and young. This study, like several others, indicated that heavy drinking by pregnant women was associated with tobacco and illicit drug use. The authors concluded that birth defects were associated with the offspring of mothers who drank heavily, but not with those whose mothers consumed moderate quantities of alcohol. The Boston researchers also noted that in some instances the 'Fetal Alcohol Syndrome' appeared to have a greater connection with marihuana (cannabis) use than with that of alcohol (Hingson *et al.* 1982; Hingson 1983). The Boston study has also produced evidence related to drinking patterns (Rosett *et al.* 1983; Weiner *et al.* 1983), the reduction of alcohol consumption during pregnancy (Rosett *et al.* 1980) and the provision of help and support for problem drinkers (Rosett 1977; Rosett *et al.* 1978).

The majority of women in the study by Streissguth (1976) and her co-workers were white and middle class. This investigation indicated that women who were heavier drinkers were more likely than those who were non-drinkers or lighter drinkers to have offspring with birth abnormalities (Streissguth 1976; Little 1977; Little, Streissguth and Guzinski 1981; Streissguth and Martin 1983; Streissguth, Clarren and Jones 1985; Streissguth *et al.* 1986). This study also indicated that as 'Fetal Alcohol Syndrome' children grew older they failed to catch up developmentally and remained small in height, weight and head circumference.

A considerable number of other studies were conducted and have been reviewed by Plant (1985, 1988). Broadly, mounting evidence supported the view that heavy maternal drinking and maternal drug use during pregnancy was associated with foetal abnormalities. Even so, little evidence emerged to suggest that 'moderate' or 'light' drinking produced harmful results (e.g. Kaminski *et al.* 1981; Gibson, Baghurst and Colley 1983; Suliaman, Du V Florey and Taylor 1986; Halmesmaki, Raivio and Ylikorkala 1987).

A Scottish study by Plant (1985) typifies the results of a number of recent investigations. This exercise involved a prospective study of 1,008 pregnant women. These were initially interviewed when three months pregnant. Three hundred were re-interviewed in the thirty-fourth week of pregnancy. Information on eventual pregnancy outcome was obtained in 970 cases, 929 of which culminated in live births. This study indicated that women who had imbibed ten units of alcohol or more on a single occasion during pregnancy were more likely than other women to produce damaged offspring. In spite of this, the evidence of this study indicated that low levels of maternal alcohol consumption were not associated with foetal harm. In addition, alcohol consumption appeared far less 'responsible' for birth abnormalities than did other factors. The latter included socio-economic status, maternal age, previous obstetric history, maternal height, tobacco smoking, diet, use of prescribed and illicit drugs. These results were very similar to those produced by several other studies, such as that from Boston.

The Scottish study related not to alcohol dependants, but to a 'normal' and mixed group of women. It is emphasized that most pregnant women do not drink heavily or use other psychoactive drugs heavily while pregnant. Plant (1985) found that a fifth of her respondents had not consumed alcohol since conception. Suliaman, Du V Florey and Taylor (1986), describing another Scottish study, concluded that 42 per cent of a group of 581 pregnant women had not drunk during pregnancy. Rubin, P.C. *et al.* (1986) from Glasgow reported finding that 65 per cent of a group of pregnant women abstained from drinking during pregnancy. Forrest *et al.* (1991) have described the progress of the study by Suliaman and his colleagues up to the time when the children were 18 months old. This revealed no association with birth abnormalities for those whose mothers had consumed up to 12 units of alcohol per week.

Rosett and Weiner (1984) have stated that inconsistent study results have been ignored and evidence has sometimes been cited selectively. They concluded that 'the danger of small amounts of alcohol has been exaggerated'. This view has recently been endorsed by Knupfer:

> There is a strong ideological and political movement in the USA to convince pregnant women not to drink any alcohol. An examination of the research literature on the results of drinking during pregnancy does not provide any evidence that light drinking is harmful to the fetus.
>
> (Knupfer 1991: 1063)

Plant, reviewing available evidence, reached the following conclusions:

> The profile of women who are heavy drinkers and may be more at risk of producing damaged babies is becoming clearer. They tend to be older, 25–30 years of age, with a low income or unemployed, to use tobacco and other drugs including legal substances such as prescribed tranquillizers and amphetamines and illegal drugs such as marijuana, heroin, LSD. The potentiating and addictive effect of alcohol in combination with other drugs must be emphasized. Heavy drinkers were more likely to have had an accident during the pregnancy. Their past obstetric history also often revealed a greater number of previous pregnancies and spontaneous abortions. These women in general were below average pre

pregnancy weight, did not routinely attend antenatal clinics and were more likely than the general population to have a spouse with a drinking problem. The nutritional status of these women is also worthy of note. Problem or heavy drinkers do not necessarily have a poor diet. However they often have difficulty with absorption and utilisation leading to nutritional deficiencies.

(Plant 1988: 16)

In most populations the 'Fetal Alcohol Syndrome' appears to be extremely unusual. There may, however, be exceptions. Dorris (1989) has provided a vivid personal account of this phenomenon amongst Native Americans. This description also provides evidence of the association between heavy drinking and illicit drug use, poor diet and poverty.

As stated by Rosett and Weiner (1984) it is apparent that, though heavy drinking may be harmful, the dangers of low levels of alcohol consumption have sometimes been inflated and distorted. A balanced view of available evidence has recently been provided in Britain by the Royal College of Psychiatrists (1986), the Royal College of General Practitioners (1986) and the Royal College of Physicians (1987). These bodies have noted the inadvisability of heavy drinking during pregnancy and have recommended either abstinence or strictly limited drinking during pregnancy. They have not recommended the type of warning labels which have been introduced in the USA.

As indicated by Plant (1988), younger women do *not* appear to be especially at risk in relation to alcohol-related birth damage. It has been emphasized in Chapter 2 that young people of either gender in Britain have not increased their alcohol consumption over the past decade. Rubin, P.C. *et al.* (1986) have also reported a decline in the level of alcohol and cigarette use amongst pregnant women.

The extent to which one form of 'deviant', 'problem' or 'risky' behaviour is intercorrelated with other such activities is one of the main themes of this book. This is discussed in some detail in Chapter 11. As already indicated in earlier chapters and in this chapter, heavy alcohol use is often associated with the misuse of cigarettes, illicit and prescribed drugs. Women who are drug dependent or who use drugs heavily during pregnancy certainly put their unborn children at risk. Rosenbaum has commented:

The state of pregnancy transforms the definition of addiction from a so-called 'crime without a victim' to one with a very real victim – the unborn fetus.

(Rosenbaum 1981: 93)

She also noted that babies born to heroin-dependent women were often characterized by prematurity and low birth weight. The effects of the use of heroin and other illicit drugs have been widely noted, especially in the USA. Such drug use is evident at all socio-economic levels, but is especially evident amongst socially disadvantaged women, many of whom use a variety of legal and illicit substances (Stimmel 1982; Chasnoff 1986).

Dependence on opiates by pregnant women is associated with high rates of abortion and with a variety of birth defects. Finnegan has described such problems thus:

> Obstetrical complications associated with heroin addiction include: abortion, abruptio placenta, amnionitis, breech presentation, increased need for Caesarean section, chorioamnionitis, eclampsia, intrauterine death, gestational diabetes, placental insufficiency, post partum haemorrhage, preclampsia, premature labor, premature rupture of the membranes, and septic thrombosis. About 10% to 15% cent of drug-dependent women have toxaemia of pregnancy, and nearly 50% of the women who are heroin dependent and have no prenatal care, will deliver prematurely. Many of these infants are not only born early, but also weigh less than normal infants of the same gestational age.
>
> (Finnegan 1982: 58)

The upsurge in the use of 'crack' in the USA has led to further evidence of drug effects in pregnancy. In some US urban areas over 10 per cent of pregnancies appear to have been cocaine exposed. Such exposure is associated with premature birth, fetal death and birth defects. Some of the latter resemble those associated with the Fetal Alcohol Syndrome: small head circumference and small size. In addition, cocaine-exposed babies often exhibit disturbed behaviour for 8–16 weeks after birth. (Revkin 1989). The effects of crack use during pregnancy have been described by Jabez.

> Drug damage to the baby can be physiological as well as neurological. The most common effects are extra digits, limbs missing and smaller heads, as well as a lot of shaking, crying and irritation.
>
> (Jabez 1990:19)

Shapiro (1989) has noted that some of the descriptions of crack's effects on babies have been exaggerated and that, given a healthy environment, most appear to shake off initial dependence within a month. However, if the baby continues to live in an environment where social and nutritional deprivation is the norm then the outlook is bleak (Revkin 1989).

Continuous exposure to some drugs during pregnancy may cause babies to be born physically drug dependent. Drugs such as opiates pass easily through the placental barrier and, due to the inability of the foetus to break down the drugs, levels of the opiates may reach higher concentrations than those found in the mother's bloodstream.

Symptoms of withdrawal and foetal distress may appear soon after birth. These are often of a general nature such as tremulousness, irritability, sleeplessness, sweating, vomiting, diarrhoea and in the more extreme cases convulsions.

In some instances withdrawal symptoms may be delayed if longer-acting drugs are still present in the baby's system. It is important to note that pregnant users of illicit drugs who rely on black-market supplies may be at greatest risk. This is due to the fact that supplies are often irregular, leading to the extremes of overdose and withdrawal. The resulting oxygen deprivation to the foetus may be one of the major risks to foetal health. An additional problem is the fact that black market supplies are often mixed with other substances many of which may be harmful to the developing foetus.

Heavy alcohol use and illicit drug use during pregnancy are associated with a variety of life-style characteristics and risk factors. Amaro *et al.* (1990), for example, have reported that these include exposure to physical violence.

Tobacco smoking, as already noted, is also associated with birth defects. The Royal College of Physicians have reported:

> It is now well established that smokers who become pregnant have a small increase in the risk of spontaneous abortion, bleeding during pregnancy and the development of various placenta abnormalities. . . . In New Zealand, Ireland and the United States there is something like a twofold increased risk of spontaneous abortion in women smoking 20 or more cigarettes a day, and this is quite independent of socio-economic, marital and other factors.
>
> (Royal College of Physicians 1986: 66–7)

The effects of maternal tobacco use during pregnancy have recently been reviewed by Frogatt:

> The observation that smoking during pregnancy is associated with an increase in fetal and neonatal mortality and a reduction in birthweight has been demonstrated in many studies since the association with low birthweight was first reported in 1957. The mean reduction in birthweight between maternal smokers and non-maternal smokers ranges between 150g and 250g. The increase in perinatal mortality is about 28 per cent. These effects persist after allowing for a number of possible compounding variables such as social class, maternal age, parity, maternal height and sex of the fetus. Both the reduction in birthweight and the increase in perinatal mortality increase with the average number of cigarettes smoked. A

change in the smoking habit before the end of the fourth month of pregnancy places the mother in the risk category appropriate to her changed smoking classification. Smoking in pregnancy has also been associated with retarded physical and mental development in children.

(Frogatt 1988: 24)

Recent evidence also indicates that 'passive smoking', that is maternal exposure to the cigarette smoking of other people, is also associated with lower birth weight (Martin and Bracken 1986; Rubin, D.H. *et al.* 1986). Frogatt (1988) has noted that three randomized trials on giving up smoking in pregnancy have been conducted. Two of these indicated that giving up smoking resulted in the birth of heavier babies (Sexton and Habel 1984; MacArthur, Newton and Knox 1987).

The motivations of pregnant women who smoke have been studied by Gillies, Madeley and Power (1989). These researchers concluded that the main reasons given were to relax, to calm down, enjoyment and because of boredom. Such attempted mood control was most commonly reported by older women who smoked fewer than ten cigarettes each day. Older women were also more likely than others to ascribe their smoking to 'addiction'.

Tobacco smoking, as elaborated in Chapter 3, has been declining in the United Kingdom. It is also inversely associated with socio-economic status so that a disproportionate number of women who smoke are from low-income backgrounds. The latter are particularly likely to be characterized by various social disadvantages.

The thalidomide tragedy provided an extreme example of the harm that drug use may cause during human pregnancy. It also served as a warning that some animal research may not identify, or be an appropriate model, for drug effects on the human foetus. Rubin (1987) has noted that approximately 35 per cent of women in the United Kingdom take prescribed drugs during pregnancy, though only 6 per cent do so in the first three months. Rubin concluded that there had been a marked decline in such drug use in the UK since the 1960s. Whittle and Hanratty (1987) have reported that 45 per cent of pregnant women in the USA take prescribed drugs. Some drugs appear to be relatively safe to use in moderate, controlled amounts. However, others are less safe. Whittle and Hanratty note dangers related to oral anticoagulants, anti-convulsants, certain antibiotics (not penicillins) and possibly sex hormones.

HIV AND AIDS

HIV infection and AIDS have added a new and tragic dimension to the possible hazards associated with pregnancy. As indicated in Chapter 7, the

spread of HIV infection and AIDS is associated in many areas with intravenous drug use (Strang and Stimson 1990). The perinatal transmission of
HIV infection has been reported. Curran *et al.* have noted:

Perinatal transmission could occur during pregnancy or during the immediate postpartum period. Detection of HIV in fetal tissues supports
the hypothesis that infection can occur in utero. This was supported by
the description of a dysmorphic syndrome in HIV-infected infants;
however, the existence of this syndrome was not confirmed in a controlled study. HIV transmission at birth through exposure to maternal
blood also seems plausible. In addition, case reports of three women
who acquired HIV by a transfusion given in the immediate postpartum
period and subsequently infected their infants suggest that breast-
feeding can result in HIV transmission.

(Curran *et al.* 1989: 29)

HIV-infected babies have been reported in areas in which intravenous drug
users have been HIV infected. Such locations include New York, Edinburgh
and Dundee. Paediatric HIV infection does not appear inevitably to lead to the
retention of HIV antibodies nor to the onset of AIDS.

Peckham and Newell (1990) have reported that in the USA and Europe
approximately 10 per cent of those who are HIV infected are women and 2
per cent are children. The same authors also reported that 47 per cent of
HIV-infected children recorded in Europe by the end of 1989 had mothers
who were intravenous drug users. The pattern of infection in the USA was
similar. Peckham and Newell concluded that HIV infection per se does not
appear to influence pregnancy outcome. The latter seems to be more
influenced by maternal health. At present the long-term outcome for HIV-
infected babies and children is uncertain. Even so, some authors have
reported 'antibody loss' by children who were initially HIV infected
(Lepage *et al.* 1987; Pahava, Good and Pahava 1987; Goetz *et al.* 1988).

To conclude, it is apparent that the use of alcohol, tobacco, prescribed
and illicit drugs during pregnancy does involve a risk to the unborn child.
It is often difficult to distinguish the precise effects of a specific drug, since
some pregnant women use a variety of substances. Studies suggest that over
90 per cent of pregnant women report using some over-the-counter drugs.
Luckily most pregnant women do not smoke, use illicit drugs or drink
heavily. Only a small minority inject drugs. Such risky behaviours, as
expounded elsewhere in this book, are themselves often intercorrelated
with a variety of other problems and with many complex aetiological
factors. The risks of 'moderate drinking' during pregnancy have sometimes
been grossly exaggerated. Even so heavy maternal drinking is often a
marker for a constellation of unhealthy and hazardous behaviours. These

place not only the mother but also the unborn child at risk. The use of tobacco, alcohol, prescribed and illicit drugs during pregnancy is clearly best avoided or at least minimized. Some encouraging trends have been evident in the youthful use of both alcohol and tobacco. Sadly, illicit drug use continues to rise in many countries, accompanied by the spread of both adult and paediatric HIV infection and AIDS.

9 Sexual behaviour

It is difficult to investigate private behaviour. As lamented in earlier chapters of this book, even surveys of alcohol and tobacco use are certainly biased and flawed by inaccurate self-reports and by reluctance to co-operate. Such difficulties are likely to be even more marked in relation to sexual behaviour (Bagnall 1991d).

Surveys of self-reported sexual behaviour were pioneered by the famous American work of Kinsey, Pomeroy and Martin (1948) and Kinsey *et al.* (1953). More recently, other studies have been conducted, but some of these preceded the advent of AIDS (e.g. Schofield 1973; Farrell 1978).

Humphries (1991) has noted that several studies of sexual behaviour were conducted in Britain during the 1950s. He concluded:

> These surveys, the first to really break the taboo on asking any questions about sex in Britain, contain fascinating information on sex during the early part of the century when some of the respondents were young. They provide some evidence that there was a gradual increase in the frequency of sex before marriage over the decades, indicating a growing relaxation of Victorian taboos between the 1900s and the 1950s. Eustace Chesser, for example, found that 19 per cent of married women born before 1904 had pre-marital sex; this rose to 36 per cent for those born between 1904 and 1914; it rose again to 39 per cent of those born between 1914 and 1924; and finally rose to 43 per cent for those born between 1924 and 1934.
>
> (Humphries 1991: 32)

Sexual activity during this period, as for many centuries past, was potentially hazardous. The Royal Commission on Venereal Diseases concluded that, in 1916, 10 per cent of the male population of Britain had syphilis and many more had gonorrhoea (Humphries 1991: 19). Only the introduction of penicillin during the 1940s transformed the situation by making a cure for these conditions available. It should be noted that much of the official response to 'venereal diseases' in the early decades of this century provided a preview of recent political and tabloid responses to AIDS. This early publicity was sexist in the extreme and often blamed disease transmission solely upon 'easy women', while apparently absolving their male partners from responsibility. Sadly, much recent comment on the AIDS epidemic has been equally unbalanced and bigoted.

This chapter does not attempt to provide a comprehensive review of the vast and rapidly expanding international literature on sexual behaviour. Instead, a partial and selective account is given of some of the recent evidence about sex amongst adolescents and young adults. This is related to HIV/AIDS risks and to the incidence of sexually transmitted diseases and unplanned pregnancies.

AIDS has provided the impetus for a huge upsurge in studies related to sexual behaviour. These have mainly been inspired by the need to examine the extent to which people may be at risk of HIV infection through sexual contact and by the need to monitor trends in such risk levels.

During 1987 a survey was undertaken of a random sample of the British population in the 16–24 age range (Johnson *et al.* 1989). This exercise elicited information from 780 people. The response rate for this study, 48 per cent, was low. This is a problem which predictably affects many studies on such a sensitive topic. The survey indicated that amongst those studied who were aged 16–24, 87.1 per cent of females and 70.6 per cent of males had experienced heterosexual intercourse. Amongst those aged 25–34 these proportions rose to 100 per cent and 97.5 per cent respectively.

The authors reported:

There is a markedly skewed distribution, with the majority of people reporting two or fewer partners in any time period and a small minority reporting 10 or more. The mean and median number of partners in the last 12 months reported by men were 1.1 and 1, respectively. . . and by women were 0.89 and 1, respectively.

(Johnson *et al.* 1989: 138)

Very few people, two males and three females, reported having had sex with somebody of the same gender. One female reported having been paid for sexual intercourse and 3.6 per cent of the males reported having paid for sex. It is probable that such reporting is subject to considerable concealment. Weatherburn *et al.* (1990) have reported that 90 per cent of a cohort of homosexual men in England and Wales had engaged in vaginal intercourse with females.

A telephone survey of 942 men in the 18–44 age group in Edinburgh and Glasgow indicated that approximately half of those interviewed reported having a single sexual partner in the previous five years. Seven per cent reported having had ten or more partners during that period. Older respondents were less likely than younger men to report large numbers of sexual contacts (McQueen, Robertson and Smith 1988).

The sexual behaviours of a sample of 480 white males aged 15–49 in England and Wales were examined by Foreman and Chilvers (1989). The study revealed that over half of the respondents had reportedly had sexual intercourse before the age of 18 and over 75 per cent had done so by the age of 20. The authors reported:

> Age at first intercourse tended to be lower in more recent birth cohorts and social classes III, and V. Men in earlier cohorts tended to have had fewer heterosexual partners, both regular and casual, than those born more recently, but there were no social class or regional differences in the number of partners.
>
> (Foreman and Chilvers 1989: 1137)

In this study, 1.7 per cent of those interviewed reported having had homosexual intercourse. Six per cent reported having at some time had a sexually transmitted disease, most commonly gonorrhoea or non-specific urethritis. The authors noted that comparison of their self-reports of infections with national clinical data suggests considerable under-reporting by survey respondents.

Foreman and Chilvers cited a recent analysis of the 1970 survey data collected by the Kinsey Institute (Fay *et al.* 1989). This suggested that 4 per cent of males had reported having homosexual intercourse at some time and 1.9 per cent reported such experiences 'occasionally' or 'fairly often' beyond the age of 19.

Ford (1989) has described the results of a survey of the self-reported sexual behaviour of 400 people aged 16–21 in Somerset. This study indicated that 92 per cent of respondents classified themselves as heterosexual. One per cent classified themselves as homosexual and one per cent as bisexual. The remaining 6 per cent provided no clear data. A comparison was made between rural and urban dwellers. This revealed that those in rural areas reported lower levels of sexual experience and later experience of first intercourse than did those in urban or semi-urban areas. In all areas at least one in seven of those surveyed reported having two or more sexual partners in the previous year. Five per cent of those in urban and semi-urban and 3 per cent of those in rural areas reported having had four or more sexual partners in the past year. The majority of those in urban and semi-urban areas, 71 per cent and 59 per cent respectively, reported not having used condoms during their last sexual encounters. In contrast, 51 per cent of the rural dwellers had done so.

Bowie and Ford noted ominously that the levels of sexual activity evident from the Somerset survey 'could eventually give rise to HIV prevalence rates similar to those found in Africa, i.e. 15–100 HIV antibody positive per 1000' (1989: 61). Durex reached the following conclusions from their own survey data:

> Many young people are not sexually active. However, those who are having sexual intercourse are likely to have multiple partners. Around 40 per cent of young men 16 to 20 claim to have had between two and six partners in the last year, and therefore could be at risk from AIDS and STDs. . . . Women in general claim fewer sexual partners than men – with 79 per cent having one compared with 63 per cent of men.
>
> (Durex 1990a: 7)

Several authors have reported that younger adults are more likely than older adults to have more sexual partners. For example, the UK Family Planning Research Network (1988) reached the conclusion from a survey of women attending British family planning clinics. This indicated that early first experience of sexual intercourse was associated with subsequent contact with larger numbers of sexual partners. Foreman and Chilvers (1989) cited evidence that early initial intercourse is a risk factor for cervical cancer, regardless of number of sexual partners (Rotkin 1981). Bachrach and Horn (1988) reported that, amongst US women, those who were younger reported higher levels of early sexual activity.

A Scottish survey by Bagnall and Plant (1991) examined the self-reported sexual behaviour and alcohol, tobacco and illicit drug use of 1,378 people aged 16–30 in two deprived areas of Edinburgh and Glasgow. This study indicated that only 7 per cent of those in Muirhouse in Edinburgh and 6 per cent of those in Easterhouse in Glasgow reported always using condoms with their current partners and that only similar proportions reported always using condoms during sex since they became sexually active. Muirhouse is an area in which there is a high level of HIV infection, mainly associated with intravenous drug use (Robertson 1987). Eight per cent of those interviewed in this locality reported having had sexual intercourse with somebody they believed to be HIV seropositive. The corresponding proportion in Easterhouse was 3 per cent. Only a small minority of those respondents had always used condoms during such contacts.

Three American studies which provided information about age at first sexual experience have recently been reviewed by Kahn, Kahbech and Hofferth (1988). The studies under consideration were conducted in 1969–73, 1982 and 1983. Although the three studies reviewed differed markedly in their dates and methods, a number of consistent conclusions emerged. All three indicated that, even by the age of 12, a small minority (up to 2.5 per cent) of adolescents have sexual experience. By the age of 15 this had risen to up to 4.3 per cent amongst white and from 7.3–24.7 per cent of black teenagers. By the age of 19 most teenagers were sexually experienced. The three studies differed considerably on the levels of younger sexual experience. Even so, they were consistent about levels of first sexual experience after the age of 15. Beyond this age 25 per cent of whites and 57 per cent of blacks had their first sexual experience. Racial differences in the age of sexual initiation and subsequent sexual history have been reported by several US authors. For example, Bachrach and Horn (1988) noted that premarital sexual activity was more commonplace amongst black than white women. Such differences, it is emphasized, must be interpreted with reference, not only to ethnicity, but to socio-economic status, income and many other factors. Another US survey recently indicated that 45 per cent of white and 56 per cent of other teenagers in the USA were sexually experienced (Aral and Cates 1989). Even so, the authors noted that teenagers exhibited the least consistent sexual activity as well as the highest rates of abstention following sexual experience, 38 per cent for whites and 31 per cent for others. This study emphasized the fact that those who are 'sexually experienced' are not necessarily currently sexually active.

Several studies have pointed to an association between early sexual experience and other 'problem' or 'deviant' behaviours. This linkage is discussed further in Chapters 10 and 11. Adolescents who are delinquent or who come from poor families have been noted to be especially likely to have early sexual experiences (O'Reilly and Aral 1985). The sexual experience of 1,255 US delinquent adolescents was examined by a questionnaire survey (Weber *et al.* 1989). This investigation revealed a very early mean age of first sexual intercourse, 13 years. Even so, the authors reported that such experience had rarely preceded puberty. The survey indicated that early sexual activity was more commonly reported by boys than by girls. A quarter of the females reported sometime having been forced to have sex compared with only 2 per cent of the males. Altogether 82.3 per cent of the adolescents surveyed reported having had sexual intercourse. Eight per cent reported that they had not had intercourse and 9.5 per cent failed to respond. The authors concluded:

> Each year after age 12 years, roughly 15–20% more females reported sexual intercourse up to age 16, when nearly 80% reported being sexually experienced. Only 3.3% of our females reported coital activity before age 10 years. . . . Eight of the ten instances were attributed to forced sex.
>
> (Weber *et al.* 1989: 399)

The relationship between high risk sexual behaviour and other factors amongst US adolescents was further investigated by Biglan *et al.* (1990). These authors concluded that 'risky behaviours' were intercorrelated. High risk sexual behaviour was associated with alcohol, tobacco and illicit drug use, together with antisocial behaviour. A variety of social variables were also associated with risk-taking. These included friends' risk-taking, 'family availability', parental support and the use by friends of alcohol and illicit drugs. Such correlations are discussed further in Chapter 11.

A British study examined some of the characteristics of teenage girls who had become pregnant. This showed that these young women were especially likely to have divorced parents, mothers who had married under 21 and whose first children had been conceived outside marriage. In addition, three-quarters of the pregnant teenagers reported having first had sexual intercourse before they were 16. Almost half of those surveyed reported that their pregnancies were unplanned and over half had failed to use any form of contraception during their initial sexual experience. These pregnant teenagers did not differ from the local population in respect of their socio-economic backgrounds (Curtis, Lawrence and Tripp 1988).

The relationship between early sexual experiences with other adolescents and later sexual behaviour and adjustment has been examined by Leitenberg, Greenwald and Tarran (1989). This study, which related to college students in the USA, indicates that such precocious experience had no discernible impact on subsequent sexual adjustment.

Prostitution, or the exchange of sexual services for money or other payment, frequently involves young people. Commercial sex, though illegal or semi-legal in many countries, is extremely widespread and involves millions of people worldwide as sellers and far more people as clients (Plant, M.A. 1990).

A study of the sex industry in Edinburgh concluded that most of those surveyed who were selling sexual services were young. Amongst females the mean age was 26 and amongst males (rent boys) the mean age was 23. This study indicated that, while most of the male and female prostitutes interviewed requested clients to use condoms, a minority did not. Approximately a quarter reported sometimes charging clients more for unprotected sex. In addition, most of the prostitutes did not always use condoms with their non-paying partners (Morgan Thomas 1990). Survey data elicited from a group of 209 sex industry clients in the same city confirmed the extensive demand for unprotected sex. The age range of these clients, most of whom were males, was 18–60 (Morgan Thomas *et al.* 1990). This study emphasized the difficulties of adopting condom use with an established partner. In addition, the relative 'bargaining positions' of partners and/or clients clearly plays a major role in influencing decisions to use or not to use condoms or to engage in risky activities. As noted by Barnard and McKeganey (1990) in relation to Glasgow adolescents, condom use is frequently rejected on a variety of grounds, ranging from discomfort to embarrassment. It has also been noted that most intravenous drug users do not use condoms with non-paying sexual partners. As in the case of the non-paying sexual partners of those in the sex industry some of these individuals are themselves drug injectors or have many other sexual partners (Donoghoe, Stimson and Dolan 1989; Morrison 1991; Klee *et al.* 1990, 1991). Des Jarlais and his colleagues in the United States have also noted the low levels of condom use evident amongst drug injectors and their non-paying partners. They have suggested that condom use may present far greater problems with established than with new partners (Des Jarlais and Friedman 1988). Intravenous drug users, though a very small minority of the population, are crucial influences upon the possible transmission of HIV infection through (mainly heterosexual) sexual contact. The relationship of psychoactive drug use and 'risky sex' is discussed in Chapter 10.

An interesting comment on adolescent sexuality has been provided by Donovan (1990). This review pointed out that children reach puberty earlier than before:

> When Johann Sebastian Bach was alive the voices of young boys dropped at a mean age of 17.7; they now drop at 13.5. Secondary characteristics in boys, including voice drop, occur late in puberty so fertility develops even earlier – at a mean age of 12.5. (Likewise, girls now experience their first menses at 12.5 with ovulation occurring two years earlier.)
>
> (Donovan 1990: 1026)

The falling age of physical sexual maturity certainly increases the emotional and behavioural pressures associated with sexual drives. Some of the adverse consequences of adolescent sexual activity have also been identified by Donovan:

> In 1969 there were 6.9 births per 1000 among 16 year olds in Britain, but in 1986 the rate had risen to 8.7, a total of 9144 live births. In 1988 some 3568 legal abortions were performed among under 16 year olds and 17,928 among 16–19 year olds resident in England and Wales. In 1985, 3,908 positive cervical smear tests were recorded among women aged under 25, compared with 1,149 in 1975.
>
> (Donovan 1990: 1026)

Donovan noted that social attitudes to adolescent sexual maturity vary markedly. In some countries, such as Pakistan (where 73 per cent of

15–19-year-olds are married), early marriage is accepted and encouraged. Elsewhere, such as in Japan, China and some African countries, abstinence is encouraged. In relation to Britain, Donovan commented that there are few strong advocates for sexual abstinence amongst adolescents. Donovan pointed out some of the factors which may influence youthful sexual development:

> One in three children will see their parents divorce before they are 16, and others will experience physical, sexual, or emotional abuse. Children who experience little affection at home may search for it through sexual contact or conceiving a baby.
>
> (Donovan 1990: 1026)

Du Rant and Saunders (1989) examined some of the possible correlates of contraceptive risk-taking amongst a sample of sexually active adolescent females in the USA. This study found no association between such risks and sexual age, religious attendance and post-menarchal age. Even so, contraceptive risks were found to be inversely associated with coital frequency and number of years of dating.

It has recently been noted that both unplanned pregnancies and abortions have been rising in Britain (Royal College of Obstetricians and Gynaecologists 1991).

THE IMPACT OF AIDS

The origins of the Acquired Immune Deficiency Syndrome (AIDS) remain unclear. Since the existence of this syndrome was recognized in the late 1970s it has become evident that the main modes of transmission of the Human Immunodeficiency Virus (HIV) are through sexual contact or through sharing infected injecting equipment. This chapter has deliberately focused upon recent, that is 'post-AIDS', studies of adolescent sexual behaviours.

The issue of AIDS has been very widely publicized in most industrial countries. Sadly, this appears, as yet, to have had only limited impact on people's behaviours. The studies described earlier in this chapter indicate that unprotected sex remains the norm amongst heterosexual adolescents and that the potential for widespread HIV transmission is high. This conclusion has already been indicated in relation to surveys such as those by McQueen, Robertson and Smith (1988), Johnson *et al.* (1989), Bowie and Ford (1989) and Bagnall and Plant (1991).

There has been strong 'consumer resistance' to safer sex and condom use messages associated with campaigns to prevent the spread of HIV infection and AIDS. Kegeles, Adler and Irwin (1988) monitored the sexual activities of a sample of sexually active adolescents in San Francisco during a year when AIDS publicity was at a high level. This study produced depressing results. The authors concluded that, on the one hand, condoms were widely perceived as having a role in preventing sexually transmitted diseases. Yet, in spite of this, sexually active adolescents continued to have multiple sexual partners and failed to increase their condom use markedly. The authors concluded:

> In our sample, males believed that their partners wanted them to use condoms, whereas females were mildly negative regarding their partners using condoms. Likewise, females were uncertain about males' desires regarding condom use when, in reality, males were quite positive about it.
>
> (Kegeles, Adler and Irwin 1988: 460–1)

This conclusion suggests, firstly, that many teenagers find it difficult to discuss sex. Secondly, some enter into sexual relationships when they know very little about their partners.

A British survey of pregnant women and girls indicated no change in sexual behaviours to reduce HIV risks. The study covered a period during which the public was targeted by several high profile AIDS campaigns (McGarry 1989). It must be noted that the study group, being pregnant, were not necessarily typical of females in general.

During the initial years of the AIDS epidemic marked changes were noted in the sexual behaviour of gay men. Specifically it appeared that there was a reduction in 'high risk' activities such as unprotected anal sex.

The changing sexual behaviours of homosexual males in England and Wales have been examined by Project Sigma. Weatherburn *et al.* (1991) have reported that condom use amongst gay men was 'relatively high'. Moreover, condom use appeared to be more commonplace with casual partners and with non-exclusive partners than with long-term monogamous partners. Even so, Hunt *et al.* (1991), reviewing data collected by the same project, concluded that earlier evidence of an increase in 'safer sex' practices had been reversed. There was a rise in the proportion of men engaging in anal intercourse between 1988 and 1989. The authors noted:

> Anal intercourse seemed to be an infrequent occurrence for a comparatively large number of them and not restricted to a small group who had yet to adopt or who had abandoned practising safer sex.
>
> (Hunt *et al.* 1991: 506)

As outlined above, available evidence indicates that intravenous drug users are still generally practising unprotected sex. As a group such individuals appear to have been much less responsive to the threat of AIDS than have gay men. The latter, it should be noted, are frequently much better educated and lead very different lives from dependent intravenous drug users, many of whom have multiple problems and are socially very disadvantaged.

Evidence about the general adolescent response to AIDS is mixed. Sonenstein, Pleck and Ku (1989) found that US survey data on young males indicated a 15 per cent rise in sexual activity between 1979 and 1988. At the same time this study indicated a doubling in the use of condoms during most recent sexual encounters. These authors reached the following conclusion:

> The young men in the sample were very knowledgeable about how the human immunodeficiency virus is transmitted, and over three-quarters of the sample did not dismiss the disease as uncommon, nor did they think that using condoms to prevent the spread of AIDS was too much trouble.

(Sonenstein, Pleck and Ku 1989: 152)

These results were more optimistic than those of many other studies. However, even this survey showed that nearly a quarter of respondents had used no contraceptive method, or no 'effective' method. Overall, 57 per cent had used condoms during their last sexual intercourse.

Several studies have noted that young survey respondents report having reduced their risk behaviours in response to HIV and AIDS (e.g. Seltzer, Rabin and Benjamin 1989). Nevertheless, it is clear that some teenagers continue to engage in unprotected sex and to have numerous sexual partners.

Balassone (1989) conducted a prospective study into contraceptive use amongst adolescents in contact with a family planning clinic service. This investigation revealed that ceasing to use contraceptive pills was associated with the belief that their behaviour involved a low risk of pregnancy and poor problem-solving skills. The youthful perception of risk is crucial to the occurrence of potentially damaging behaviours. This is discussed further in Chapters 11 and 12. Beliefs and behaviours are not necessarily consistent. A recent British study obtained information from fifty-six sexually active adolescent girls in a juvenile assessment centre or attending a genito-urinary medicine clinic. This revealed that, while most of these girls recognized the dangers of HIV infection and some were concerned about these, they had done little to minimize their risks (Clarke, Abram and Monteiro 1990).

SEXUALLY TRANSMITTED DISEASES

There has been a marked change in the patterns of sexually transmitted disease in the United Kingdom since the 1960s. Syphilis, relatively rare, has undergone a slight decline. Gonorrhoea increased during the 1960s and early 1970s, but has subsequently declined. In contrast, non-specific genital infections and genital warts have increased considerably. There has also been a rise in genital herpes. Trends in the numbers of new cases of such diseases between 1968 and 1986 are depicted in Figure 9.1.

The first authenticated case of HIV infection in the United Kingdom *appears* at the time of writing to date back to the 1950s. AIDS was,

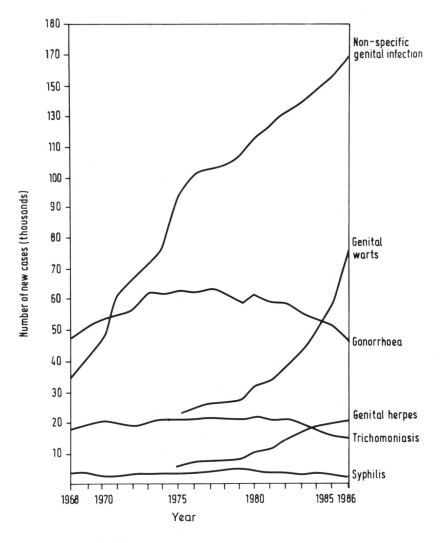

Figure 9.1 Sexually transmitted diseases (United Kingdom 1968–86)
Source: McMillan 1991

however, not formally recognized until much later. Trends in the number of recorded cases of AIDS and AIDS deaths in the United Kingdom are shown in Figure 9.2.

As this figure indicates, the number of such cases had risen from 750 in April 1987 to 4,568 in April 1991. More than half of the cumulative total of cases during this period had died. It is emphasized that this does not mean that half of those cases identified each year die during the same year.

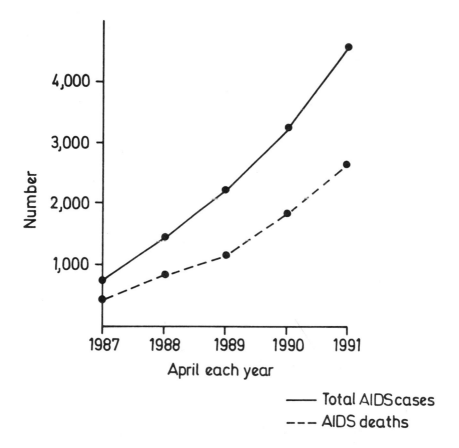

Figure 9.2 AIDS cases and AIDS deaths (United Kingdom 1987–91)

Source: Department of Health 1991

SEX IN THE AGE OF AIDS

A long-running London show was entitled *No Sex Please, We're British.*
The evidence reviewed above would suggest that the implication of this
title is highly inaccurate. Adolescents, in Britain, the USA and elsewhere,
are often sexually experienced and sexually active. There is evidence to
suggest that younger adults are, if anything, more sexually active than their
predecessors. Early sexual experience appears to be commonly unprotected
and often associated with other forms of problem or risky activity. Surveys
of adolescent AIDS awareness indicate that *general* levels of knowledge
are high but that some people also have major misconceptions. In the
United Kingdom such misconceptions have been fostered by bizarre dis-
information by some of the tabloid media. The latter have reinforced the
totally erroneous view that HIV/AIDS are really risks only for gay men or
drug injectors. A recent survey by Gillies (1989) indicated that four out of
five 14-year-olds were not worried about AIDS.

As the evidence cited in this chapter indicates, adolescent sex remains,
even now, commonly unprotected by condoms. So far, behavioural responses to the AIDS epidemic have, outside the gay community, been
extremely limited. Moreover, as indicated by Weatherburn *et al.* (1991), the
move to 'safer sex' noted some years ago amongst gay men may have
dissipated to some extent.

Adolescents, as already remarked, mature earlier now than ever before.
This, as noted by Grant and Demetriou, poses serious problems:

> Developmentally, adolescents reach physical maturity before they are
> cognitively able to appreciate the consequences of their behavior. A
> teenager's primary source of information regarding sexuality is his or
> her peer group, all of whom are experiencing and reinforcing the same
> behaviors. The family, the major socializer of other behaviors, is not as
> powerful a force in shaping responsible sexual behavior because of
> parental discomfort with sex education and sexual discussions. This is
> the result of a social milieu in which sex is frequently portrayed but
> rarely linked with responsible behavior or accurate, non-judgemental
> information.
>
> (Grant and Demetriou 1988: 1286)

The frightening reality is that providing people with AIDS information
does not, by itself, influence behaviour. The reduction in high risk sexual
activity noted amongst gay men followed the intrusion of high levels of
HIV infection and AIDS into their communities. It may be that general risk
reduction will not occur until catastrophic levels of HIV infection become
established throughout the sexually active population. It is emphasized that

current 'normal' sexual practices are well able to engender such levels of infection. This cannot be blamed upon any identified sub-group in the population regardless of what the tabloid press print. Galt, Gillies and Wilson (1989) have described the results of a survey of 766 19-year-olds in Doncaster. This indicated that, although levels of HIV-related knowledge were high, few people believed that they were at risk of HIV infection themselves.

The AIDS risk perceptions and sexual behaviour of people attending a sexually transmitted disease clinic have been examined by James, Gillies and Bignell (1991). This study showed that only 19 per cent of these individuals perceived themselves to be at risk of HIV infection. The least aware of HIV/AIDS risks were the young who also had poorer knowledge of HIV-related issues.

CONDOM USE

Between 1986 and 1987 British condom sales rose by a remarkable 20 per cent. This increase was attributed to publicity about AIDS. Durex, the major UK condom manufacturer, noted that subsequent increases in condom use were much smaller. Durex reported:

> this recent increase in condom sales partly results from HEA advertising campaigns. Another reason for the increase in condom usage has to be the improved purchase availability of condoms. Not only are more outlets now prepared to retail condoms, but the in-store displays are currently larger than ever before thereby encouraging self-selection. In addition to this, there has been a significant increase in the number of condom vending machines, including units sited in female toilets . . . this actively appears to have been effective amongst younger people, who are, of course, sexually maturing against an AIDS back cloth and as such have a different attitude towards condom usage than previous generations of teenagers.
>
> (Durex 1990a: 2)

This report noted that almost 25 per cent of the UK population aged 15–55 had used condoms in the past three months. Condoms were the main form of contraception reportedly used by males, especially those under the age of 20. Condom use was particularly popular amongst younger people and those living in the South of Britain. Amongst those aged 16–20, 35 per cent had used condoms in the past three months. Amongst those aged 21–25 the corresponding proportion was 31 per cent. Beyond that condom use decreased with age. It was noted that only 73 per cent of males who were classified as using condoms as their main mode of contraception had used condoms in the past three months. Durex noted that this could be attributed either to failure to engage in sex or 'an aptitude to practise unprotected sex'. In view of some of the evidence noted earlier in this chapter the latter interpretation appears to be reasonable. This study revealed that only 17 per cent of condom users regard such devices solely as contraceptives. Nearly three-quarters perceived condoms as having both contraceptive value and acting as protection against AIDS and other sexually transmitted diseases.

Young single people were those most concerned about AIDS. Amongst these aged 16–20, 21 per cent reported being very worried and amongst those aged 21–25 the corresponding proportion was 16 per cent. Fifteen per cent of males and 10 per cent of females reported being 'very worried' about their personal AIDS risks. Forty-eight per cent of respondents aged 16–20 and 41 per cent of those aged 21–25 claimed to have changed their sexual behaviours because of the threat of AIDS. These apparently positive findings need to be set against the following conclusion:

> It was also encouraging that usage of condoms with a new partner increased from 4% of the sample to 5% following the advertising [this refers to a Health Education Authority advertising campaign].
>
> (Durex 1990b: 10)

This statement, coming years into the AIDS epidemic, is chilling. The increases in condom use are, of course, good news. Even so, most young people do not at present use condoms and few use them routinely. Durex (1990a) noted that approximately two-thirds of those aged 16–25 did not use condoms.

It should be noted that before the advent of AIDS the pill had become a popular form of contraceptive amongst young women. The pill, though a reliable contraceptive, does not provide protection against sexually transmitted diseases or cervical cancer. Condoms do serve such a protective role. A combination of AIDS publicity, as noted above, and more widespread information on the risks of the contraceptive pill have led to an increase in condom use to the extent that it is now British young people's preferred form of contraceptive. Durex (1990a) have recently reported that: 'the condom is still seen as the method for people who have a large number of partners, not in steady relationships, and used by young people'. Survey data collected for Durex indicated that condoms are perceived as the best mechanical protection against sexually transmitted diseases.

The evidence presented in this chapter is mixed and is generally far from reassuring. A substantial proportion of young people continue to have multiple sexual partners and the bulk of the sexually active population has made few concessions to the arrival of HIV and AIDS. As recently emphasized by Gillies and Carballo (1990), available international evidence suggests that many people have extremely misleading and inaccurate perceptions of their personal HIV risks. Even the initial behaviour changes by gay men appear to have been at least slightly dissipated with the passage of time. Some intravenous drug users, amongst whom high levels of HIV infection have been noted, have certainly reduced their risk-taking behaviours. Even so, it is emphasized that such have only been lowered and by no means eliminated. All of this suggests that HIV infection will continue to spread throughout the sexually active population. Such infection threatens to move from an epidemic to an endemic phenomenon.

10 Alcohol, drugs and risky sex

Porter . . . and drink, sir, is a great provoker of three things.
Macduff What three things does drink especially provoke?
Porter Marry sir, nose-painting, sleep and urine. Lechery sir, it provokes, and unprovokes; it provokes the desire, but it takes away the
performance: therefore much drink may be said to be an equivocator
with lechery.

Macbeth II, iii

The use of alcohol and other psychoactive drugs is deeply intertwined with
social behaviour. As indicated by earlier chapters, drinking, smoking and
illicit drug use all become increasingly commonplace as young people
grow older. In addition, the use of licit and illicit drugs is widely viewed as
a hallmark of attractiveness, maturity and sociability. Because of the highly
social nature of much of their use, alcohol and other drugs are frequently
associated with sexual behaviour. Psychoactive drugs are associated with
sexuality for two broad reasons. The first of these is the cultural and social
connections between the use of such substances and sexual encounters.
Very often drinking or other types of drug use may simply be the conventional accompaniments or precursors of dating and sexual activity. The
second reason is that drugs have and are widely believed to have effects
upon sexual arousal and performance.

Ridlon has made the following comments on a historical example of
beliefs about alcohol and sex:

From the beginning of civilization there has been a connection between
drinking and involvement with sex. Wine drinking by women was
punishable by death in early Rome because it was linked directly to
adultery. It was feared that if a woman opened herself to one male vice,
drinking alcohol, she might open herself to another, sexual promiscuity.

(Ridlon 1988: 27–8)

The complexity of the relationships between drinking alcohol and sexual behaviour has been ably delineated by Leigh:

Alcohol may be a symbolic instrument of courtship or an agent of physical incapacitation that enables men to take sexual advantage of them [*i.e. women*]. Controlled research on the effects of alcohol on subjective and objective physiological arousal in women is rare, and more is needed to explain the puzzling findings produced so far. Alcohol increases women's subjective sexual arousal, but this increased desire does not necessarily lead to initiation of sex. A woman's intoxication might, however, increase the likelihood that she will be seen by a male partner as sexually available. Liberal sexual habits are correlated with liberal drinking habits, but an understanding of the causal order underlying this relationship is elusive.

(Leigh 1990a: 141)

RISKY SEX

Intoxication has long been connected with failure to use condoms and with sexually transmitted diseases and unplanned pregnancies (e.g. Flanigan and Hitch 1986). In spite of this, very little 'research interest' appears to have been focused on this linkage before the advent of AIDS. There are, however, some notable earlier studies which have considerable relevance to this issue, such as the classic study by Cavan (1966) entitled *Liquor License: An Ethnography of Bar Behavior*. Other relevant works include *Drugs and Sexuality* by Soloman and Andrews (1973) and the important work *Drunken Comportment: A Social Explanation* by McAndrew and Edgerton (1970). As noted by Cavan and more recently by McKirnan and Peterson (1989) a variety of drinking settings, such as bars, have clearly defined sexual identities and functions. The connection between psychoactive drug use and sexual behaviour has gained greatly added relevance because of the steadily spreading AIDS epidemic.

Central to concern about the role of drug use in general in relation to AIDS risks is the concept of 'disinhibition'. This has already been referred to in Chapter 5 in relation to alcohol and crime. Essentially this, in a sexual context, suggests that people may be less inhibited if under the influence of alcohol or other psychoactive drugs. Robertson has commented:

In the presence of appropriate environmental cues the effects of alcohol may be misattributed or transferred to sexual arousal. Expectancies regarding the effects of alcohol on sexuality as well as subjective arousal, bear a curvilinear relationship to dosage. These expectancies are similar for men and women and vary as a combined result of social learning and personal experience. They function as personal and social attributions of feeling, thought and behaviour related to alcohol.

(Robertson 1990)

Stall and his colleagues provided a spur to other research by reporting that 'high risk' sexual activity amongst gay men in the USA was associated with the use of alcohol, amyl nitrite (poppers), cannabis and other drugs (Stall *et al.* 1986; Stall 1988; Stall and Ostrow 1989). This work indicated that there was a clear increase in unprotected or risky sex if such activity was combined with psychoactive drug use. Stall (1988) reported that men who used drugs with sex were at least twice as likely as other men to engage in risky activities. A Scottish study of young people who had married while teenagers revealed a similar association. Fifty-eight per cent of males and 48 per cent of the females in this study reported having consumed alcohol immediately prior to their first experience of sexual intercourse. Males who had drunk before intercourse were more than three times less likely than those who had not done so to have used some form of contraception, 13 per cent and 57 per cent respectively. The corresponding proportions of females were 24 per cent and 68 per cent (Robertson and Plant 1988).

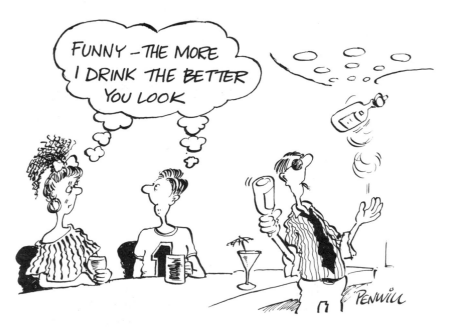

Figure 10.1 Disinhibition

Source: Roger Penwill

Hingson *et al.* (1990) carried out a telephone survey of teenagers in Massachusetts. The investigation indicated that heavier drinkers and cannabis users were 2.8 times and 1.9 times less likely respectively to report using condoms during sex. Unlike the earlier surveys by Stall *et al.* and Robertson and Plant, the study examined whether alcohol and other drug use influenced *individual* behaviours. This is important since the associations noted earlier might simply imply that some people are generally predisposed to take risks. If this is true then such people's use of alcohol or other drugs may not affect their risk-taking behaviour. Hingson and his colleagues found that amongst their respondents who were drinkers or illicit drug users 16 per cent reported using condoms less after drinking and 29 per cent reported using condoms less after illicit drug use. A second survey by Hingson, Strunin and Berlin (1990) re-examined the alcohol use and sexual behaviour of teenagers in Massachusetts. This study indicated that amongst sexually active 16–19-year-olds, 61 per cent had engaged in sexual activity after drinking and 13 per cent reported being less likely to use condoms under such circumstances.

Parker, Harford and Rosenstock (1990) have described some of the results of the sixth phase of the US National Longitudinal Study of Youth which was carried out in 1984. This showed that 'sexual risk taking' was associated with alcohol and drug use amongst both males and females.

As noted in Chapter 9, Plant, Plant and Morgan Thomas (1990) examined alcohol, illicit drug use and sexual activity amongst a non-randomly selected study group of male and female prostitutes in Edinburgh. This indicated that many were heavy drinkers and that illicit drug use was widespread. More than 75 per cent of the men and women interviewed reported at least sometimes drinking while contacting clients. The majority had at least sometimes used cannabis or other illicit drugs while working. In addition, these respondents estimated that more than half of their clients were under the influence of alcohol and that approximately a third were under the influence of illicit drugs. These findings reflected the fact that many of those included in this study contacted clients in bars, discos, hotels, clubs or other licensed premises.

A second Edinburgh study group of 'sex industry clients' were interviewed during 1988 and 1989. These were 206 males and three females who had at some time paid for physical sexual services. The majority, 78.3 per cent, of those individuals reported drinking at least sometimes while making contact with prostitutes. Over 40 per cent reported that drinking was the norm on such occasions. In addition, 29.5 per cent reported at least sometimes using illicit drugs when contacting prostitutes. Self-reported condom use was not related to alcohol use amongst the male clients of female prostitutes. Even so, those rent-boy clients who had drunk the most were the least likely to use condoms (Morgan Thomas, Plant and Plant 1990). It is notable that the self-reports of these clients were, to a high degree, consistent with those obtained from prostitutes in the same locality.

Mott and Haurin (1988) have described the results of a survey of young men and women in the USA. This examined connections between sexual activity and alcohol and illicit drug use. This study showed no link between earlier sexual experience and first use of alcohol and drugs. However, individuals who became sexually active later were more likely to have commenced alcohol and cannabis use around that age. The authors noted a closer link between cannabis use and sexual activity than was evident in relation to alcohol use and sex:

> This is consistent with the idea that marijuana use may be a less accep-table type of behavior in early adolescence than is the consumption of moderate amounts of alcohol.
>
> (Mott and Haurin 1988: 135)

The study concluded that heavier alcohol use, being a more 'deviant' activity, may be expected to be more closely linked with adolescent sexual activity than casual drinking.

Flanigan *et al.* (1990) have reported several studies indicating that women view alcohol as an aphrodisiac and that women frequently drink prior to sexual intercourse, including their first experience of intercourse. Flanigan *et al.* further concluded, from a study of forty-three instances of unplanned pregnancy, that these were precipitated by a number of factors:

> Alcohol and drug use, then, while not necessary or sufficient to deter a woman from protecting herself against pregnancy, may be a significant element amongst other causal factors.
>
> (Flanigan *et al.* 1990: 213)

A follow-up study by Plant, Peck and Samuel (1985) has been cited in earlier chapters. During 1988 and 1989 the original study group was sought for a fourth phase of this follow-up study. These individuals were then aged between 25 and 27. Three-quarters of the original respondents were suc-cessfully re-interviewed. The relationship between their alcohol consump-tion and sexual behaviour was examined. Alcohol consumption levels in general were not related to self-reported condom use. Even so, both males and females who reported a high frequency of combining sexual activity with alcohol consumption were seven times less likely than other respon-dents to use condoms during vaginal intercourse. In addition, females who had experienced higher levels of adverse alcohol-related consequences were more likely than other women to report that they regarded their sexual behaviour as 'risky'. Males who had experienced higher levels of adverse alcohol-related consequences reported having had more sexual partners in the previous year than did other males (Bagnall, Plant and Warwick 1990). The authors noted that the majority of respondents in this study had had only a single sexual partner in the previous year. Accordingly, much more information is required to determine levels of 'AIDS risks'. The latter depend, not only upon specific sexual behaviours, including levels of condom use, but the precise sexual histories of those involved, their sexual partners and the histories of these partners. Such factors need to be related to the overall extent and distribution of HIV infection in particular localities. It should, however, be noted that Edinburgh is an area with a high rate of identified HIV infection, mainly associated with intravenous drug use (Strang and Stimson 1990).

Ford's study in Bristol was cited in Chapter 9. This indicated that most of those surveyed reported that alcohol consumption made them less sexually inhibited and made sex more pleasurable. In addition, most of the males and a large minority of females reported that drinking made them more likely to forget about HIV/AIDS risks and pregnancy. Sixty-four per cent of males and 50 per cent of females stated that they were less likely to use condoms after drinking. Ford noted that older respondents were especially likely to view alcohol as leading to fewer sexual inhibitions. He commented:

> This finding may indicate the effect of a longer social learning in which sexual interaction is increasingly associated with social situations in which alcohol is consumed.
>
> (Ford 1989: 72)

The study indicated that alcohol was perceived by these young adults as having a greater association with sexual behaviour than had cannabis. It was concluded that 'those respondents who consume the highest levels of alcohol perceive the drug as having considerable influence on their sexual feelings'.

Temple and Leigh (1990) have described a Californian general population study in which adults were asked for details of their most recent sexual experiences and also their most recent sexual experiences with a new partner. This investigation indicated that encounters with new partners were more likely to involve alcohol consumption. Even so, drinking per se was not associated with risky sex.

Leigh (1990a, 1990b) has described this and two other US investigations. The study groups were 117 volunteers who kept diaries of their drinking habits and sexual activities, 844 respondents from a San Francisco mail survey and respondents involved in a household survey of Contra Costa County in California. Drinking was unrelated to risky sex amongst gay men. This finding contrasts with that reported by Stall and his co-workers. Amongst heterosexuals drinking was only associated with risky or unprotected sex amongst females in the San Francisco mail survey who had consumed five or more drinks. Conversely, drinking was weakly associated with *safe* sex amongst males and females in the diary study. The latter, it should be noted, were not in any sense a representative group of people. These results, like those elicited by Bagnall, Plant and Warwick, do not suggest that drinking by itself is necessarily or invariably associated with risky sex. Leigh further noted the following:

> risky sexual behaviour was *not* related to the *proportion* of sexual activity involving drinking and *was* related to the *proportion* of sexual activity involving cocaine and other drugs in gay men only. Frequency of risky sex in heterosexuals was predicted largely by total frequency of sex, with small amounts of variance contributed by frequency of sex with a partner who was drinking or using drugs.
>
> (Leigh 1990c: 199)

Temple (1991) has reported evidence from a US prison study. This also indicated a connection between combining alcohol and sex with risky sex.

The connection between high risk sexual activity and drug use amongst gay men has also been noted in relation to a New York study described by Siegel *et al.* (1989).

Several authors have recently noted the possible role of crack in relation to unprotected sex. Fullilove *et al.* (1990) have described a study of US crack users. This indicated high levels of sexual activity while under the influence of crack. The authors noted that, in some areas, such as San Francisco, females sometimes exchange sexual favours for supplies of crack. The authors further reported that some individuals appear to be very 'passive' in relation to sexual precautions:

> What is not clear, however, is how such passivity is causally related to crack use and sexual behavior. Is the passive style induced by the drug and by participation in crack culture, or does it precede use of the drug and involvement in the culture?
>
> (Fullilove *et al.* 1990: 367)

McEwan *et al.* (1991) conducted a postal survey of 1,388 students in North East England and a quota survey of 3,000 university students. This study indicated that drinking was associated with a failure to use contraceptives, having sex with 'a person who would not usually be chosen' and contact with more sexual partners. Heavier drinkers of either sex were more likely than other respondents to have had three or more sexual partners, to have had unprotected sex or to have had sex with 'a promiscuous person' in the past year. The authors concluded: 'Alcohol is associated with unsafe sex in a young, predominantly heterosexual population' (1990: 1). McEwan and his colleagues also found that sexual risk-taking was associated with tobacco smoking. They concluded: 'Both smokers and non-smokers who were heavier drinkers, however, took more sexual risks than their lighter drinking peers' (1990: 8).

The association between high risk sexual behaviour and psychoactive drug use has been further endorsed by a US study of adolescents conducted by Biglan *et al.* (1990). This investigation showed that risky sex was intercorrelated with cigarette smoking, alcohol and illicit drug use. It has been noted that unprotected sex was commonplace amongst those who are alcohol dependent (Windle 1989). In addition, a high rate of HIV infection has been noted amongst inner-city alcohol-dependent people in the USA (Scheifer *et al.* 1990).

To summarize, several, but not all, studies have indicated that alcohol and other drugs may be associated with risky sex, amongst both adolescents and older people. As noted by Strunin and Hingson (1991), the evident associations between heavy drinking and risky sex could reflect a variety of other factors. These include personality, situational and behavioural influences. Strunin and Hingson also noted that 'adults are more likely than adolescents to be married or to have steady sexual partners which could influence their sexual practices after drinking or drug use'. These authors have commented that the relationships between psychoactive drug use and sexual behaviours need not be static. They cited US evidence that amongst gay men reductions in both drinking and risky sex occurred over time.

The relationship between alcohol and sexual behaviour is influenced by people's expectations of what effects alcohol might have on sexual activity. Leigh's (1990b) mail survey of households in the San Francisco area, found that males and females, both heterosexual and homosexual, differed in relation to their sex-related alcohol expectancies. Gay males and lesbians reported stronger expectancies for decreased nervousness and increased sexual riskiness than did heterosexuals. Heavier drinkers were especially likely to endorse the view that alcohol would influence sexual behaviour. Leigh concluded:

Those with stronger beliefs about alcohol's ability to cause decreased nervousness about sex or enhance sexual experience were more likely to drink in conjunction with sexual encounters, and, if drinking, were more likely to drink larger amounts. This relationship was particularly strong for individuals who were nervous and/or guilty about sex. In addition, sex-related alcohol expectancies were related to some of the behaviors and feelings inherent in sexual encounters, such as that respondents with strong beliefs about the ability of alcohol to decrease nervousness were more likely to initiate sexual activity.

(Leigh 1990b: 925)

The still questionable role of alcohol in relation to sexual activity has been emphasized by Gillies:

> It could be argued, therefore, that alcohol use is simply a marker for high risk-taking behaviour and that disinhibition effects from alcohol are secondary, at least in gay men. . . . . On balance data published recently would appear to suggest that alcohol consumption in itself may not in fact be strongly related to unsafe sexual behaviour. . . . . It may, however, be more commonly associated in individuals who have a higher risk profile in general.

(Gillies 1991: 3)

Sexual arousal is in itself a powerful form of disinhibition. The recognition of a 'risk' is not in itself enough to deter people from indulging in potentially hazardous behaviour. Alcohol, illicit drugs and sexual behaviour are all appealing for a variety of potent reasons. They can be enjoyable, exciting, confer status and are socially approved, especially by young people's peers. Research into the association between alcohol, illicit drugs and risky sexual behaviour is continuing. Available evidence has produced conflicting results, though several studies have supported the conclusion that 'high risk' sex is *associated* with drinking and other forms of drug use. This connection, as emphasized by Strunin and Hingson (1991), certainly reflects other factors. Moreover, decisions about sexual activity, as noted by Morgan Thomas (1990), are influenced by the relative 'bargaining positions' of the partners with or without drugs. Human behaviour can, however, be modified and there has, as described in Chapter 9, been some evidence of increased condom use by young adults in some areas. The subject of problem prevention or, more realistically, harm reduction is the subject of Chapter 12.

To conclude, on balance available evidence supports the view that there is an *association* between alcohol, certain other drugs and risky sex. Even so, a clear causal connection has not yet been demonstrated and further research is required to provide additional clarification. It is probable that this will remain a thorny area of research. Some people doubtless use alcohol and other drugs for sexual purposes, being influenced by both popular and obscure beliefs and misconceptions about their disinhibitions or alleged aphrodisiac properties. In addition, some people, whether drunk or sober, are probably more inclined to take risks than others. This issue is considered further in the next chapter.

11 Risk-takers

It is a basic conclusion from the evidence reviewed in this book that there is nothing inherently 'deviant' or 'abnormal' in the use of psychoactive drugs. Most people do use such substances. While the actions described in this book all involve possible adverse consequences, the majority are essentially normative and familiar. The reason they are matters for concern are because they are widespread. The greater the use of drugs and the more frequent the sexual encounters, the greater the risk of misuse. The 'official' view, as propounded by health professionals, researchers and policy makers, is that heavy drinking, the use of tobacco and illicit drugs and unprotected sex are all risky.

However, after decades of publicity about adverse consequences, over a quarter of the adult British population continue to smoke, millions drink too much and use illicit drugs. In addition, though a decade into the AIDS epidemic, most sexual encounters continue to lack the simple protection provided by condoms. Why is this? Are humans inherently suicidal or stupid? Do we not know about the risks to which we constantly expose ourselves? The answers are far more complex than these questions would suggest. Even if a particular risk is acknowledged, people are understandably inclined to weigh their personal chances of experiencing adverse consequences. Most individuals would rightly conclude, for a variety of reasons, that their risks are acceptable. Young people, often at their physical peaks, typically view themselves as invulnerable. When tragedies happen to people, others often rationalize to reinforce the view that 'it will never happen to me'. This rationalization is just as normal amongst drinkers, smokers and drug users as it is amongst racing drivers or mountaineers. A notable feature of such rationalization has been identified by Davies (1991). This is that when a person overcomes a risk this is typically attributed to individual prowess, such as bravery or skill. If the risk ends in disappointment, even tragedy, this will frequently be ascribed by the protagonist to 'bad luck' or to external factors. Others, however, may ascribe such accidents and failures to incompetence, poor judgement or other personal flaws.

To a degree risk is synonymous with excitement and sensation-seeking. Some types of risks are perceived, not as folly or sin, but as praiseworthy and remarkable. Sporting activities provide an excellent example of a form of risk that is widely viewed as admirable. The distinguished mountaineer Chris Bonington has described such activities thus:

> To me adventure involves a journey, or sustained endeavour, in which there are the elements of risk and of the unknown which have to be overcome by the physical skills of the individual. Furthermore, an adventure is something that an individual chooses to do and where the risk involved is self-imposed and threatens no-one but himself.
>
> (Bonington 1981: 13)

There are, of course, different levels of risk. Some activities are inherently far more dangerous than others. It is possible to indulge to a modest, and relatively safe, extent or to take repeated and major risks. As indicated by Chapters 2, 3 and 4, most of those who use alcohol, tobacco and illicit drugs do not become heavy, chronic or 'problem' users. Most young adults in Britain do *not* drink heavily and use neither tobacco nor illicit drugs. Those who are 'professionally concerned' with health and social problems may weigh risks in epidemiological or 'objective' terms. Ordinary people, that is the vast bulk of humanity, probably use different criteria by which to assess their vulnerability to risks. In particular, it appears that people are influenced, not necessarily by the 'reality' of a risk, but by what they *perceive* that risk to be.

The perceived (or more accurately, imagined) invulnerability of teenagers has been described as the 'Personal Fable' (Elkind 1967, 1984, 1985). Elkind suggested that the Personal Fable can be positive and productive as well as potentially damaging. This is because it may inspire adolescents to aim for exceptional goals, which some in fact do manage to attain. On the negative side of the balance, the Personal Fable may motivate individuals to ignore 'reasonable precautions' such as the use of contraception during sexual encounters. More recently Jack has stated:

> If the healthy role of the Personal Fable is to assure adolescents that they are special and unique . . . they may use it to enhance self-esteem. . . . The Personal Fable might protect self-esteem by allowing adolescents to believe that they can perform a risky act without experiencing the negative sequelae. Rather than 'lose face' in front of peers, risky behaviour might be undertaken since the Personal Fable would prevent a realistic appraisal of the consequences.
>
> (Jack 1989: 336)

Jack also noted: 'Risk-taking and experimentation during adolescence are considered normal behavior because they help adolescents achieve independence, identity and maturity' (1989: 337). In spite of this, Jack concluded, such risk-taking is associated with the major causes of mortality amongst adolescents, such as accidents, often attributable to the youthful assumption of personal invulnerability. She also noted that adolescent pregnancies are frequently fostered by a belief in personal immunity from adverse consequences.

Another view of the possible value of risk-taking for adolescents has been provided by Irwin and Millstein:

Risk-taking in middle and late adolescence serves to fulfil developmental needs related to autonomy as well as needs for mastery and individuation. The pursuit of new activities and practice taking initiative are positive attributes that can lead to both negative and positive outcomes. Mastery needs are frequently met by experimentation, which often involves testing limits and taking risks.

(Irwin and Millstein 1986: 86S–87S)

Irwin has stated that: 'risk-taking is a normal transitional behaviour during adolescence' (1989: 124).

Human behaviour often fails to oblige social scientists or other researchers by conforming meekly to sweeping and often over-simple theories. The complex aetiology of many behaviours makes it unlikely that specific activities, such as alcohol, tobacco or other drug use, can be explained by or reduced to a single theoretical perspective. Risk-taking provides a good example of a multi-faceted phenomenon which is not easy to explain and which (as elaborated in the next chapter) is difficult to modify, let alone prevent. Available evidence, some of which has been described in this book, suggests two broad empirical conclusions. Firstly, risk-taking, to varied degrees and in different forms, is extremely widespread, to the extent that, as Jack has affirmed, it is normal amongst adolescents (as well as amongst older people). Secondly, the pattern and extent of particular risks taken clearly varies amongst different sub-groups of the population and between different social, cultural, ethnic and national groups. Young Scots are far more likely to drink heavily (or at all) than are young Saudis. Young Austrians are more likely to die in mountaineering accidents than are young Nigerians. The reasons for such variations in local patterns and traditions of leisure, sport and other forms of risk-taking are obvious. As already emphasized, risk in itself need not be deviant or abnormal. Even so, the pattern of such behaviours is far from uniform. Jessor and Jessor (1977) produced an important book in which they propounded 'Problem Behaviour Theory'. This is an essentially psychological

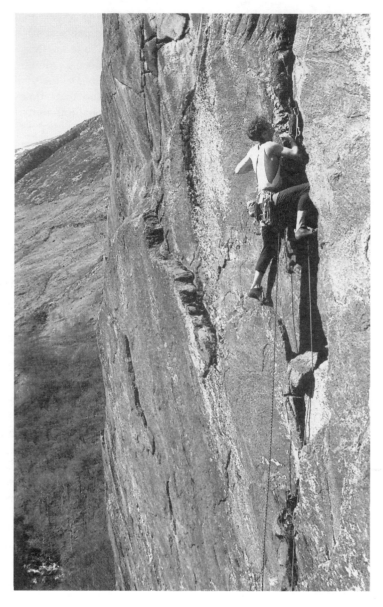

Figure 11.1 Acceptable risk? Craig Smith climbs Conscription (Glen Nevis)

Photograph by Noel Williams

perspective. It advances the view that the disposition to engage in 'problem behaviours' such as heavy drinking, illicit drug use or unprotected sex is influenced by biographical and social-psychological variables. Such influences include personality, beliefs and the behaviours which are approved of by significant others (Jessor 1987). The implications of this theory are profound and have great relevance for consideration of risk-taking. Jessor and his colleagues have reported, on the basis of extensive empirical studies in the USA, that adolescent problem behaviours are interrelated (Donovan and Jessor 1978; Jessor *et al.* 1980; Jessor and Jessor 1984; Jessor *et al.* 1991).

> Overall the empirical evidence supports the existence of organized patterns of adolescent risk behavior. These structures of behaviors, taken together, reflect an adolescent's way of being in the world. . . . Part of the answer probably lies in the social ecology of adolescent life, an ecology that provides socially-organized opportunities to learn risk behaviors together and normative expectations that they be performed together.
>
> (Jessor 1991: 9)

Jessor suggests that risk-taking is, by definition, entwined with life-style. He, like other commentators, also states that risk has both positive and negative aspects. He suggests that a reformulation of risk requires an audit of its costs and benefits. Many risk behaviours have positive consequences, at least in the eyes of those who engage in them. Conversely Jessor has commented:

> in too much discourse in this field there has been a failure to recognize the fundamental role of socially-organized poverty, inequality, and discrimination in producing and maintaining a population of at-risk youth.
>
> (Jessor 1991: 1)

An important review, *Children Under Stress*, noted the connection between emotional problems amongst young people and a variety of social factors. These included illegitimacy, adoption, parental separation and social deprivation (Wolff 1970). Such backgrounds, it was noted, were associated with youthful psychiatric disorders, delinquency and precocious or risky sexual behaviour. In addition, Wolff concluded that such patterns of problems were sometimes transmitted from one generation to the next.

Youthful behaviours are thus associated with the behaviours or characteristics of their parents. Jessor, Donovan and their associates have emphasized that those born into socially disadvantaged circumstances are likely to be 'at risk' in multiple ways. Such 'transmitted deprivation' has been noted by many researchers. It is not only those from deprived backgrounds who may be influenced by their parents. Green *et al.* (1991)

concluded from a cohort study of young people in Scotland that the alcohol consumption of daughters from non-manual backgrounds was positively associated with that of their parents.

A study of French-speaking adolescents in Montreal examined risk-taking activities such as heavy drinking, smoking and seat belt use. This indicated that adolescents from intact families reported lower levels of such risks than did adolescents whose parents were divorced or separated (Saucier and Ambert 1983). As noted by Greydanus:

> The adolescent population is the only age group in America with an increasing mortality rate during the past 25 years. Violence remains the leading cause of adolescent deaths, with accidents, suicides, and homicides accounting for more than 75 per cent of teenage mortality. Substance use contributes to this phenomenon, as in the high fatality rate of adolescents who drink or use marihuana and drive. Many of these risk taking behaviors, in fact, are interconnected and have their origins in such diverse factors as childhood experiences, parenting, peer-pressure, timing of puberty, self-esteem, depression, ethical and religious training, and education.
>
> (Greydanus 1987: 2110)

Jonah (1986) reviewed evidence on the possibility that drivers aged 16–25 had greater 'accident risks' than older drivers. This review indicated that some people are especially predisposed to engage in several forms of risky behaviour in relation to driving. For example, Evans, Wasielewski and von Buseck (1982) reported that drivers who do not wear safety belts are especially likely to drive close to the vehicles in front of them. Jonah suggested that future research should examine the possible connections between a variety of health-risk behaviours. He suggested that attempts to change a single form of health risk may be ineffective since other forms of risk might simply be adopted as substitutes.

Goldbaum *et al.* (1986) concluded from a US survey that failure to wear vehicle safety belts was associated with other forms of risk-taking behaviour. In particular, seat belt use was inversely associated with smoking and heavy drinking, and was associated with being overweight and in-active. Olenckno and Blacconiere (1990) examined some of the correlates of seat belt use amongst university students in the USA. This investigation revealed that illicit drug use, smoking status and sex were significant predictors of whether or not students wore safety belts while driving. In addition, alcohol use and drinking and driving were also inversely as-sociated with seat belt use. The authors reached the following general conclusion: 'The findings appear to support the hypothesis that failure to wear seat belts is part of a general pattern of risk taking behaviour among young people' (1990: 161). They cited other studies which had linked failure to wear seat belts with tobacco smoking (Eiser, Sutton and Wober 1979; Cliff, Grout and Machin 1982; Grout *et al.* 1983). Jonah concluded that young drivers *do* take more risks than older people. He commented that the role of alcohol in youthful traffic accidents remained unclear: alcohol could be either a *cause* or a *correlate* of such occurrences.

> Young drivers generally have a poorer risk perception than older drivers ... evidence that does exist suggests that risk has a greater utility among youth primarily in the expression of emotions like aggression, the seeking of peer approval, the facilitation of feelings of power and control and the enhancement of self-esteem. Moreover, there is some evidence that youth tend to underestimate the disutility of risk (e.g. being killed in an accident). This might be a function of young people's perception of themselves as invincible. Death is a very remote event for most young people.
>
> (Jonah 1986: 268)

Further evidence linking youthful drinking and driving with other 'problem behaviours' has recently been described by Klepp and Perry (1990). These authors, from a survey of 1,700 US students, found that a variety of personality, perceived environmental and behavioural factors were associated with drinking and driving. These factors included alcohol and cannabis (marihuana) use, risk-taking behaviour and family structure.

A recent US study by Neubauer (1989) indicated that health risk-taking was weakly associated with seat belt use and smoking. These results emerged only amongst individuals who reported that their health was good for people of their age. The author concluded that 'poor health status and dogmatism may contribute to denial of risk and risky sexual behaviour' (1989: 1255). Hingson, Howland and Winter (1989) have reported that people who ride with drunken drivers are themselves heavier drinkers and are more likely to engage in risky behaviours than other people. This finding emphasizes the importance of peer pressure and social norms in reinforcing potentially dangerous or unhealthy behaviours.

The relevance of risk-taking to certain types of sporting activities has already been mentioned in this chapter. Young (1990) examined sensation seeking and criminality amongst a small study of student athletes and non-athletes. He discovered that sensation seeking was associated with self-reported criminal behaviour amongst the student athletes, but not amongst other students. Student athletes were more likely than the control group of non-athletes to report interest in a variety of risky activities. These included climbing, parachute jumping, drinking, 'partying', gambling and sex. They also reported a distaste for repetitive tasks.

As already noted, a considerable body of evidence supports the view that several 'risky behaviours' are associated. As described above, such behaviours include the use of alcohol, tobacco and illicit drugs, sexual behaviour, traffic safety and 'health behaviours'. The work of Richard Jessor and his associates has already been noted. Jessor and his colleagues, as outlined above, have propounded the view that not only are 'problem behaviours' frequently inter-correlated, they also signify a lifelong career of disposition to move from one form of problem behaviour to another (e.g. Jessor and Jessor 1977; Donovan and Jessor 1978). 'Problem Behaviour Theory' was related to prospective studies of cohorts of adolescents in the USA. The theory hinges upon the concept of 'proneness' to engage in risk or 'problem' behaviours (Jessor, Donovan and Costa 1990). These authors note modest but significant correlations between a number of personality measures, health behaviours and problem behaviours amongst adolescents. In addition, co-variations between problem behaviours have also been reported to be evident amongst young adults (Donovan and Jessor 1985; Donovan, Jessor and Costa 1988).

The work of this group reinforces the complexity of the issues surrounding youthful behaviours. These need to be weighed and considered from social and psychological as well as from purely behavioural perspectives.

Available evidence sustains two broad conclusions, both of which have major implications for the prevention of harm. Firstly, risk-taking is natural, commonplace and, in some form or another, inevitable. Secondly, while most young people can be expected to take some risks, a variety of potent factors foster and often perpetuate risky or problem behaviours. On the basis of current information it appears that there is considerable overlap between one form of risk-taking and others. Risks are often interconnected. Different studies produce varied results and these would appear to support the view that young people may move into and out of different styles and degrees of risk. Risk-taking is closely associated with life-style. People seek excitement in all manner of ways. For some, especially those in derelict inner-city areas, the most obvious and accessible routes might be through the crack house or the syringe. For others, the same status, experience and meaning are obtained with the hang-glider, the skis or the ice axe and the rope. At a different level, while some people actively participate in risky pursuits, others derive vicarious excitement or additional reinforcement by watching or reading about them (e.g. Burroughs 1959; Simpson 1988).

This chapter, and indeed this book, does not consider the issue of what motivates people to take risks. The issue of motivation is, of course, crucial to the understanding of risk-taking. From even the limited evidence cited above it is a reasonable deduction that risks result from strong psychological drives for many and probably for most people. If this is so then, from a health perspective, it is important to consider and to investigate whether or not the reaction to such drives can be modified. It is of equal importance to discover the extent to which, if certain forms of risk-taking are effectively reduced, other risks are adopted as alternatives.

12 Prevention and harm minimization

The provision of counselling, support or clinical management is beyond the scope of this book. Even so, attention is now focused on the issues of either preventing or minimizing the harm associated with the various forms of 'risk-taking' discussed in earlier pages. In particular, these risks relate to the use and misuse of alcohol, tobacco and illicit drugs or to unprotected sexual activity.

The evidence presented above supports a number of conclusions which have major implications for prevention or harm minimization. These include the following:

* Risk-taking is commonplace adolescent behaviour.
* The use of legal and, to a lesser extent, illicit drugs is very widespread. Most adolescents use some form of drug regularly by the time they are 15 or 16.
* Youthful sexual activity has been little affected by the risk of HIV/ AIDS.
* Risky behaviours are fostered by a variety of powerful factors. Most of these are difficult to counter.
* Different people in different social positions are subject to different influences.
* Adolescents typically perceive themselves as being invulnerable to harm.
* Intervention strategies should take into account the ways in which young people perceive at least some risks as prestigious.

PREVENTING THE YOUTHFUL MISUSE OF ALCOHOL AND OTHER DRUGS

As outlined in Chapters 2–7 the use and misuse of legal and illicit drugs amongst young people is extremely widespread. Luckily most drug use is relatively moderate and does not involve chronic, heavy or dependent use.

In spite of this it is evident that all forms of psychoactive drug use, however popular and generally harmless, even beneficial, have a negative side. Whenever a drug is widely used some people will take it in an inappropriate or damaging way. There is no neat mathematical formula, but it is apparent that whenever the overall level of substance use (e.g. alcohol, tobacco, illicit drugs) rises or falls, so too does the level of drug-related adverse consequences. Accordingly, levels of drug-related harm do reflect the extent to which specific substances are in general use. The latter is influenced by a host of social, psychological and political and economic factors. Such considerations not only dictate the legal status of particular drugs, but also influence the ways that are deemed appropriate to curb or prevent 'drug problems'. Traditionally, problems related to legal drugs have been approached in far less sweeping or draconian ways than those associated with illicit or socially disapproved drugs. The latter have been regarded as targets for total elimination, rather than as being suitable for 'controlled' or 'moderate' use. Alcohol, tobacco and illicit drug control policies are highly politicized since strong moral fervour, massive public health costs and major economic considerations are involved in the formulation and application of such policies (Bruun, Pan and Rexed 1979; Taylor 1984; Davies and Walsh 1983; Freemantle 1985; Henman, Lewis and Malyon 1985; Grant 1985). Drug control policies are also beset by one major dilemma: the drugs that cause the greatest harm are those that are legal, socially approved and most widely used and esteemed. The latter, due to their very popularity, are by far the hardest to contain and the least likely to be tackled by rigorous control policies. The fate of Prohibition in the USA or, more recently, of attempting to curb vodka consumption in the former USSR underlines the fact that, to be viable, control policies need to have public support (Bakalar and Grinspoon 1984).

Drug control policies may be dichotomized into those intended to reduce demand and those intended to restrict supply.

DEMAND REDUCTION

The ideal solution to drug misuse would be if it was possible to prevent people from using drugs in a damaging manner. Strategies to achieve this goal, as noted above, have been strongly influenced by the legal status of specific drugs in specific locations. Alcohol, though legal and widely used in most countries, is proscribed in others. Tobacco is generally legal while the opiates are generally illegal. Accordingly, demand reduction policies have tended to aim towards the restricted use of legal drugs while enjoining the complete avoidance of substances which are banned.

There is a vast literature on health education designed to curb the misuse of alcohol, tobacco and illicit drugs. Many educational initiatives have been conducted with little reference either to the education research literature or to the practical realities that influence drug use behaviours. Strunin and Hingson (1991) have noted that explanations of risky behaviours amongst adolescents have sometimes used models and theories such as the Theory of Reasoned Action (Fishbein and Ajzen 1975), Social Learning Theory (Bandura 1984) and the Health Belief Model (Janz and Becker 1984). The Theory of Reasoned Action has been discussed earlier in this book. This theory suggests that people's behaviour is influenced by a wish to seek approval and by what individuals perceive as their friends' and significant others' wishes. Social Learning Theory advances the view that behaviours are influenced by the consequences of one's past actions and the observed consequences of the actions of others. Strunin and Hingson commented that self-efficacy is important in this context since it influences individual confidence and perceived competence to avoid risks and to influence significant others to do the same. The Health Belief Model implies that individuals balance the perceived merits and disadvantages of specific behaviours. Such an assessment is clearly influenced by knowledge of health and related issues. Other theories of health behaviour exist. Bagnall (1991c) has drawn attention to the importance of individual, pharmacological, social and environmental factors in influencing drug-related behaviours. Such influences have been elaborated further in Chapter 1. Tones (1987) has propounded the Health Action Model. This notes the importance of factors which deter healthy behaviours. Such barriers include social beliefs and misconceptions and public policies.

As noted earlier in this book, many powerful forces work to counter health education in relation to legal and illicit drugs. Sadly, available evidence on the effectiveness of past alcohol and drug education makes depressing reading. Dorn has stated that 'no known method of drug education can be said to reduce drug use' (1981: 281). This sombre view is supported by an extensive array of evidence. Major reviews of alcohol and drug education have reached broadly consistent conclusions (Kalb 1975; Kinder, Pape and Walfish 1980; Schaps *et al.* 1981; Bandy and President 1983; Coggans *et al.* 1989; Bagnall 1991c; May 1991). These authors have inferred that those education initiatives which have been evaluated (and most have not) have been ineffective. Some have even been counterproductive. In addition, it has been suggested that young people who are better informed about illicit drugs may regard the latter, not as more dangerous, but as being safer (Glaser and Snow 1969; Swisher 1971). Pickens (1983) has suggested that drug education is likely to be irrelevant .if provided before young people are interested or involved in drug use. If it follows such use, it is likely to be ineffective.

Available evidence supports the simple conclusion that providing young people, or others, with information on alcohol, drugs or other health-related issues does not necessarily (or even probably) lead to behaviour change. Moreover, the use of fear-arousing or 'horror film' approaches is clearly unproductive and should at all costs be avoided. Human beings, as indicated in Chapter 11, are not wholly rational. The concept of 'Personal Fable' was discussed in the previous chapter. This is important since the message of many health education initiatives is severely undermined by the widespread adolescent belief in personal invulnerability (Elkind 1967, 1984, 1985).

The news is not all bad. Some studies have produced more encouraging results. It is evident that health education can increase levels of factual knowledge, even though the impact of such changes on behaviour is unpredictable.

Thomson (1978), reviewing tobacco education, concluded that, while most initiatives had proved disappointing, some success had been achieved by individual counselling and the provision of smoking withdrawal clinics. McAlistair *et al.* (1981) reported that high school students in California were trained, with a degree of success, to stand up to peer pressures to drink, smoke and use illicit drugs. In addition Aaro *et al.* (1983) and Gillies and Willcox (1984) have reported positive results from tobacco education initiatives. The latter study in England produced evidence that health education in schools did deter 9–11-year-olds from beginning to smoke. Gillies, Pearson and Elwood (1986) have also reported that 15–16-year-olds who recalled having received tobacco education were less likely subsequently to have begun to smoke than teenagers who did not recall such education.

Bagnall (1991c) designed and assessed the utility of an alcohol education package for use in schools with teenagers. Her study indicated that some modest behaviour benefits were produced by this inexpensive and 'user friendly' initiative. She assessed her results, and available evidence, in these terms:

We may be on the road to success, but at the same time we are becoming more aware of the complexity of the task. There are no easy answers, and there is little doubt that much hard work awaits researchers, teachers and all who work with young people.

(Bagnall 1991c: 108)

Although cigarette use is increasing world-wide there have been marked falls in tobacco use in some industrial countries, including Britain and the USA. Such falls reflect a number of factors such as recession, price and health awareness (Godfrey and Robinson 1990; Maynard and Tether 1990).

The Royal College of Physicians (1986) concluded that British anti-smoking campaigns had produced short-lived effects, but did serve to increase public awareness of a serious health problem. The decline in cigarette use in Britain has certainly been aided by product price rises, together with several decades of clear-cut public information.

EXHORTATION? JUST SAY 'NO'

In many countries the rise of illicit drug use, especially amongst urban adolescents, has led to heightened, even exaggerated concern. Such 'moral panics' frequently accord undue weight to problems which are far from new and which are often endemic rather than fresh epidemics (Cohen 1972). A frequent political response to such concerns, real or imagined, is to mount high profile mass media campaigns. During the past decade several of these have been conducted in Britain. The most notable of these were the 'Heroin Screws You Up' campaign in England and Wales and the 'Don't Die of Ignorance' campaign on AIDS (which was conducted on a UK basis). The latter is discussed later in this chapter.

It is sometimes important to distinguish between an educational campaign and an exercise in exhortation or propaganda. Education is usually taken to involve increasing awareness of factual knowledge. Exhortation or propaganda may involve the provision of factual material but may also advise or attempt to convey a specific message. The latter was exemplified by the view that heroin users become sick and pathetic:

> Take heroin and before long you'll start looking ill, losing weight and feeling like death. So if you're offered heroin, you know what to say. HEROIN SCREWS YOU UP.

Campaigns of this type appear to be largely prompted by a political assumption that they are popular and that they convey a sense of 'official determination' to rid the planet of a particularly nasty scourge. Initiatives of this type in several countries have been launched to the accompaniment of ringing declarations that the particular problem will be eliminated completely. Events tend to prove otherwise. The 'Heroin Screws You Up' campaign has already been very widely discussed and severely criticized (*British Medical Journal* 1985; Plant 1987). Such campaigns have little to commend them. They simply do not deter people from using drugs. 'Heroin Screws You Up' was an extreme and notorious example of the type of publicity used much earlier in the twentieth century to combat sexually transmitted diseases. The campaign did not have the support of many researchers, clinicians, drug agency workers or health educationalists. Like many other expensive public ventures, it contained some extremely dubious messages and was not evaluated in a competent or credible way (Marsh 1986). Accordingly, the impact of this campaign remains unclear. Newspaper reports suggested that some of the supposedly unattractive pictures of heroin users were adopted as teenage pin-ups. At least one journalist interpreted the results of the campaign as indicating an *increase* in heroin use. Fear arousal is an inferior method of health education.

AIDS CAMPAIGNS

The obvious seriousness of AIDS has prompted a remarkable level of international action to curb the spread of the virus through unprotected sex or through sharing infected injecting equipment. As indicated in Chapter 9, British mass media publicity about AIDS led to a 20 per cent increase in condom sales between 1986 and 1987 (Durex 1990a, 1990b). This was a notable advance, but, sadly, falls far short of the types of changes that are needed to prevent HIV infection becoming as widespread as syphilis and gonorrhoea were in the United Kingdom until the 1940s. A high profile public-funded mass media campaign on AIDS was mounted throughout the United Kingdom. This campaign was accompanied by a torrent of AIDS-related publicity, dramas, discussion and general coverage. The 'official campaign' adopted a formula reminiscent of the much earlier public initiatives related to syphilis. As during the already then thoroughly discredited 'Heroin Screws You Up' campaign, fear was adopted as one of the key ingredients. This is illustrated by Figure 12.1.

This campaign, with images of tombstones, icebergs, and gravesides, aroused widespread alarm. Large numbers of worried but healthy people sought HIV tests, but the numbers of those being identified as HIV infected were not influenced by the campaign. This expensive exercise, in so many ways a repetition of the ill-famed heroin venture, was widely criticized by health professionals and AIDS specialists. One of the latter has since commented that the United Kingdom alone in Western Europe chose to use fear as the key to its national AIDS campaign. An evaluation indicated that during the period of the campaign (which included all households receiving AIDS information leaflets) levels of AIDS-related knowledge increased as did *lack of* sympathy for people with AIDS. Only a fifth of those surveyed reported having used a condom during their last sexual encounters. Even so, 46 per cent of the 16–17 age group reported using a condom on this occasion. No evidence of behaviour change emerged (Department of Health and Social Security/Welsh Office 1987).

More recent, lower key public campaigns including local initiatives have been directed at more specific target groups, notably intravenous drug users. These are exemplified by Figure 12.2.

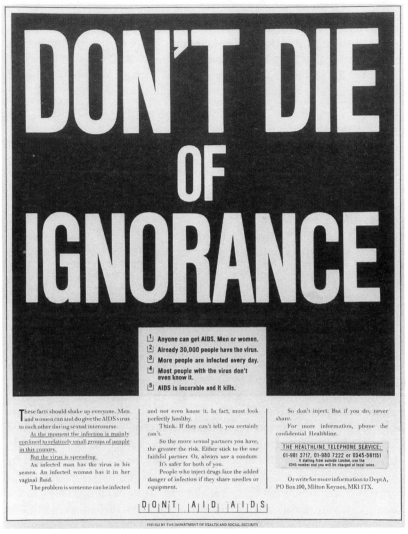

Figure 12.1 Don't die of ignorance

Source: HMSO

The tone of such national campaigns has been in contrast with a more positive approach adopted in several local initiatives. The latter are exemplified by Lothian Region's 'Time to Take Care' Campaign.

As discussed in Chapter 9, available evidence shows that, although general levels of AIDS knowledge in the United Kingdom are reasonably high, there has been only a very muted behavioural response to AIDS. Most

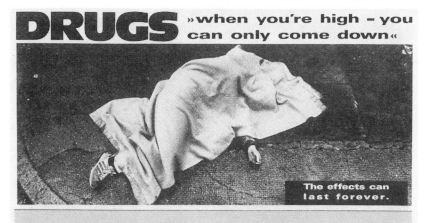

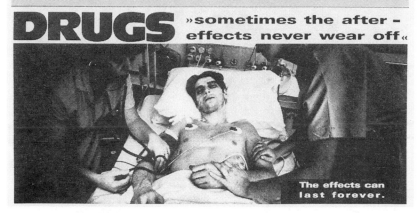

Figure 12.2 1990 drug campaign

Source: HMSO

people continue, for a variety of reasons, not to see themselves as being at risk. It is clear that public exhortation is not, in itself, an effective means of bringing about a reduction in life-threatening or unhealthy behaviours. The slogan 'Just Say No' has been widely applied in Britain, the USA and elsewhere in relation to public anti-drug campaigns. One African country recently conducted a poster campaign which adapted this to proclaim 'Just Say No to Sex'. This exhortation implies, if anything, an even greater degree of optimism than was required to apply this message to drug use. Slogans of this type are simply empty rhetoric since they totally fail to account for the forces which impel people to engage in behaviours which are both completely normal and yet at the same time often potentially risky.

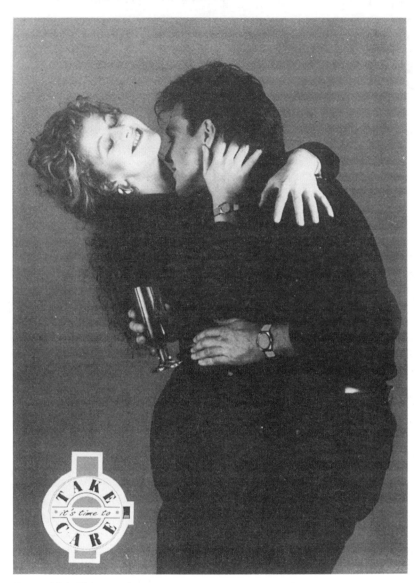

Figure 12.3 Time to take care

Source: Lothian Regional Council

Available evidence is extremely depressing. The present pattern of hetero-sexual behaviour amongst young people in Britain is quite compatible with the eventual spread of HIV infection up to the levels already evident in Uganda and some other African countries. This grim prospect is certainly possible since sexually transmitted diseases have already, only a few decades ago, reached comparable proportions in the United Kingdom. The majority of gay men have radically changed their sexual behaviours, but did so only when confronted by the reality of infection, illness and death. Is the rest of the population to be unaffected until forced to witness, on a much more enormous scale, the same catastrophe? This seems certain to be not only Britain's but the world's greatest health challenge for the foreseeable future.

HARM MINIMIZATION: A LIGHT AT THE END OF THE TUNNEL?

So far this chapter has not been cheerful. There is scant evidence that it is possible to prevent young people misusing alcohol, using illicit drugs or engaging in unprotected sex. In spite of this, clear progress has been made in some countries, but not world-wide, in discouraging youthful cigarette use. Some marginal improvements have also been noted in relation to youthful willingness to use condoms. A wide variety of strategies have been adopted to achieve reductions in risky or health-threatening behaviour. As noted in Chapter 5, the British are now markedly less likely to drink and drive than they were a decade ago. These are heartening developments to which few would object. Unfortunately, illicit drug use and AIDS have inspired a number of strategies which are extremely con-troversial and to which some people object very strongly. As already emphasized, education and public campaigning are not necessarily the same things. Many past endeavours have been designed to discourage activities such as illicit drug use or risky sex. In general such strategies have produced only modest or disappointing results. There are some people who, for many different complex and powerful reasons, will continue to inject drugs or to engage in high levels of sexual activity. This obvious fact has prompted many concerned with these health issues to adopt strategies designed to minimize the harm associated with both drug use and sexual activity. Two main tactics have been adopted to reduce such risks. Firstly, there is the provision of sterile injecting equipment, or the means of sterilizing such equipment, for intravenous drug users. Secondly, the vig-orous provision of condoms has been advocated. Both strategies have stimulated strong opposition. The provision of sterile injecting equipment or enabling drug users to sterilize their own equipment has been attacked on the grounds that it condones illicit drug use, or even that it is a form of genocide. The provision of condoms has been opposed on religious grounds, because it too signifies support for immoral behaviour and for a variety of other reasons. The ethical merits and limitations of such objections are beyond the scope of this book. Public health issues invariably involve legal, moral, religious and ethical controversy. Those concerned with public health frequently have to run into conflict with powerful moral and religious forces, especially if issues of sexuality are involved (Mort 1987).

Many of those who work in the alcohol and drug problems fields have for decades attempted to minimize the damage inflicted by the misuse of these substances. 'Harm minimization' or 'harm reduction' is nothing new. Over two decades ago it became clear that some 'problem drinkers' or 'alcoholics' could successfully adopt a moderate or controlled level of drinking without returning to the tragic consequences of their heavy alcohol use (Heather and Robertson 1981, 1986). This revelation was, and even now continues to be, regarded as heretical by those who perceive 'addictions' as discrete, uniform phenomena. Similar conclusions have been reached in relation to opiate dependants, some of whom either give up drug use or eventually revert to low-level and sporadic use (Thorley 1981). Moreover, it has been standard procedure in many countries for decades for some opiate users to receive 'maintenance doses' of methadone or other heroin-like alternatives. Such maintenance has been fostered by the belief that, although this involves continued drug use, it involves far fewer risks than continued illicit injecting with its often associated criminal life-style.

The spread of HIV infection by the sharing of infected injecting equipment has been noted in Chapter 7 and has also been widely discussed elsewhere (e.g. Strang and Stimson 1990; Stimson 1991). In spite of a depressing array of legal, political and other obstacles, a number of initiatives have been launched to supply intravenous drug users with sterile injecting equipment (often given in exchange for used equipment) or to provide people with the means, such as bleach, by which injecting equipment may be sterilized. Such policies have frequently been accompanied by the provision of free condoms for intravenous drug users and the availability of non-injected methadone. Clear evidence has emerged to indicate that such approaches have had a degree of success. 'AIDS risks' amongst intravenous drug users have, in a number of localities, been reduced, though not eliminated entirely (e.g. Donoghoe *et al.* 1989; Greenwood 1990; Donoghoe 1991; Morrison 1991; Stimson 1991).

Major problems remain. Risk reduction is evident where the means to achieve it has been provided. This excludes many areas in which such strategies are now urgently needed, especially in developing countries with limited resources. Only some people respond to risk reduction strategies and many respond in a very limited way. Parallel success has been noted in relation to men and women in the sex industry in certain areas (Plant, M.A. 1990). It has been possible, through outreach work, peer education and condom supply, to much increase the use of condoms with clients (paying partners). In spite of this, both drug users and those in the sex industry (sometimes the same people) have proved resistant to using condoms with their regular partners or lovers. The latter may be a major source of HIV infection.

There probably is no magic bullet whereby the problems of alcohol, tobacco, illicit drug misuse or risky sex can completely be overcome. Nevertheless, harm minimization is possible if applied in a practical, user-friendly way to those who are most likely to be at risk. Harm minimization does not imply, as some critics have alleged, necessary support for illicit drug use, prostitution or other illegal behaviour. Some drug workers take the view that the most effective form of harm minimization is to stop injecting or, better, stop using drugs. A massive public health threat requires brisk and thorough action. Harm minimization offers a good beginning. This may involve or lead to cessation of drug use.

CONTROLLING DRUG SUPPLIES

Societies have varied views about the legitimacy of specific drugs. Substances such as cannabis, LSD, cocaine and heroin are widely banned. Even so, the use of cannabis, coca and opium is traditional in some areas. Tobacco and alcohol are in widespread legal use. In spite of this alcohol was proscribed in the USA between 1920–33 and is currently banned in several Islamic countries.

Drug use reflects supply, price, availability, demand and many other factors, as indicated in Chapter 1. It is evident that if a drug is widely used its misuse will present more of a problem than if it is only rarely used. This is as true of alcohol and tobacco as it is of heroin and cocaine. It is not surprising, therefore, that the greatest toll of drug-related harm relates to the legal and most popular substances. In industrialized countries these are alcohol, tobacco and prescribed drugs. The preceding section of this chapter has indicated that, although health education can achieve modest gains, it is not a panacea for alcohol, tobacco and illicit drug misuse. In consequence considerable attention has been paid to controlling the availability of the substances that cause such serious problems, while at the same time being so persistently in demand.

The extent to which such controls are attempted depends upon the legal status of a specific drug in a specific location. Substances such as cannabis,

LSD, heroin and cocaine are the subject of massive law enforcement or 'interdiction' activities. These are intended to eradicate supply completely. The immensity of this task has been ably described by Bruun, Pan and Rexed (1979), Freemantle (1985) and by Henman, Lewis and Malyon (1985). It is often a losing battle against world-wide demand, massive political power, economic and even military resources. In spite of the problems of such control policies, they do reduce and remove a proportion of the supply of drugs which would otherwise be available for human use.

Legal drugs are controlled in different ways. In most countries alcohol and tobacco are both legal and in everyday use. Since their use is not often in question, they are produced and distributed legally and taxed to the point of political and economic expediency. As noted in Chapters 5 and 6, the health damage associated with the misuse of alcohol and tobacco, especially the latter, is considerable. There are, for very good reasons, a number of controls on their usage, especially by young people. In the United Kingdom it is an offence to supply tobacco products to those below the age of 16. It is also illegal for those below the age of 18 to purchase alcohol in bars. In addition, liquor licensing laws and laws on alcohol-impaired driving attempt to regulate important possible areas of alcohol misuse. As indicated in Chapters 3 and 6, tobacco use in the UK has been falling. This decline has probably been facilitated, not only by new hostile social attitudes to smoking, but also by the increased price of tobacco products. Alcohol consumption has been no less price influenced, but rose from the end of the Second World War until 1979. Since then, as indicated by Figure 2.1, alcohol consumption in the UK has declined a little and remained relatively stable. Similar post-war rises in per capita alcohol consumption were also evident in the USA and in many other countries. These rises were, predictably, accompanied by a proliferation of alcohol-related problems. The public health implications of rising alcohol consumption have been elaborated by many commentators (e.g. Bruun *et al.* 1975; Central Policy Review Staff 1979). In essence it has been concluded that, since there is a clear link between the overall level of alcohol consumption and levels of alcohol misuse, to curb the latter one must control the former. There is considerable evidence to support the connection between the overall level of alcohol and tobacco consumption in a country and the levels of alcohol and tobacco-related problems (e.g. Sales *et al.* 1989). In spite of this it is emphasized that different sub-groups of the population react differently to consumption changes over time (Duffy 1991). Moreover, it is sometimes possible for specific problem levels to be moved in different directions from the *general* level of substance use. This has recently been exemplified by the major fall in the proportion of drivers and riders killed in accidents who were above the legal blood alcohol level (see Table 5.2). This fall greatly exceeds the minor changes evident in UK alcohol consumption over the period 1979–89. Fashions in the use and misuse of alcohol and other drugs may periodically change, irrespective of consumption levels. This fact offers some hope that people can become more restrained in their use of such substances. Even so, the public health perils of the steady rise in any form of psychoactive drug use are clear and provide a maze of thorny political considerations. These have been discussed further elsewhere (e.g. Grant and Ritson 1983; Maynard and Tether 1990; Godfrey and Robinson 1990).

The most popular drugs cause the most widespread problems and are the least likely, in a democracy, to be the targets of draconian control policies. Politicians, public health specialists, educationalists and social scientists often attempt to reconcile the irreconcilable or to devise strategies that control, but not to an uncomfortable degree. In consequence, measures are adopted which are high on visibility and low on effectiveness. Mass media exhortation campaigns exemplify this. Random breath testing, though having a high level of popular support, and already shown to be valuable in Finland and Australia, continues to be rejected on grounds that remain obscure, especially to the victims of drunken drivers (Peacock 1992). Local by-laws in Coventry, Dundee and Motherwell have banned drinking on the streets in specified areas (see Figure 12.4). However, it is questionable whether this really solves basic problems, or simply moves them from one area to another.

Many of the strategies introduced to make some impact on the levels of drug problems are well intentioned. Few are ever properly assessed and their effects remain unknown. Some very different problems, such as the sharing of infected syringes or drunken driving, can be influenced markedly by determined action, backed by public or political commitment. Others, such as the wish to use drugs or to take risks, are harder to solve.

Human behaviour is influenced by a host of powerful factors. Accordingly, preventing or even minimizing human health risks is an ambitious objective. From the evidence cited above it is apparent that the provision of information is not enough, by itself, to lead to behaviour change. In addition, mass media 'propaganda' campaigns with simplistic messages run the risk of being counter-productive, ineffective or at least being wrongly perceived as health education.

Health education is important, but is as yet at an early stage. Health education can achieve, and already has achieved, positive results in a number of contexts. Available evidence suggests that health education is most effective when reinforcing or being reinforced by social pressures and by extended exposure of the target group to accurate information perceived as being directly relevant to specific individuals. Campaigns aimed at the

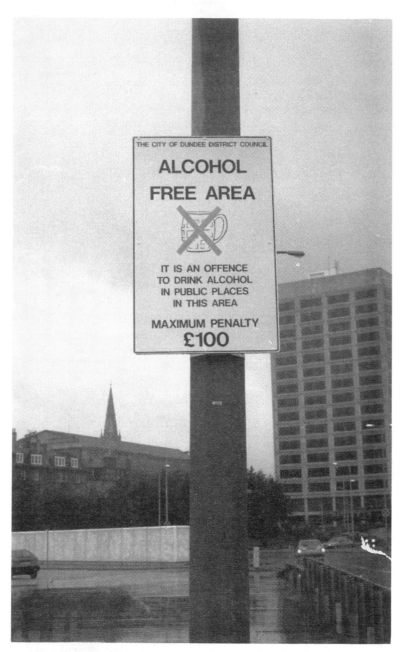

Figure 12.4 The Dundee experiment

Source: *The Courier and Advertiser*

general population have generally fallen on deaf ears because they did not appear to have such direct relevance.

It is unrealistic to imagine that the young, or their elders, are likely to give up alcohol or drug-related risks, or those associated with sexual behaviour, completely. Even so, harm minimization strategies have already achieved a reduction, if not an elimination, of risk-taking. Preventive approaches need, if possible, to have clear objectives and specific target groups. Methods should be devised in the light of past experience. Above all, such strategies need to be assessed or evaluated in order to improve future responses to important areas of human behaviour.

13 Conclusions

This book has presented an inevitably selective and incomplete picture of a number of potentially risky behaviours. A number of major conclusions emerge from this review. The first is that 'young people' are by no means the only members of the human race to expose themselves to possible harm. In certain respects the young compare well with older people. They are less likely to smoke than their parents and they are probably less inclined to use prescribed tranquillizers than are older people. Even so, from a variety of perspectives, youth, adolescence and the twenties are a time of active experience seeking. A degree of risk-taking is not deviant but normal amongst young people in all socio-economic positions.

While risk-taking is commonplace, it is evident that some people take more risks than others. This involves both a heightened degree of risk and in some cases a wider range of risks. A profusion of behavioural studies provides empirical evidence to support the conclusion that different types of youthful risk-taking or 'deviant' activity are inter-correlated. There is also evidence, as described by Jessor, Donovan and their associates, that there are connections over time between risky behaviours: some people remain risk-takers. Available evidence leads to two further conclusions. The first is that some forms of risk are associated with social disadvantage, poverty, homelessness, unemployment, bad housing, fragmented family structure and stressful life events. The connection between poverty and problem behaviours is clearly evident, not only in relation to intravenous drug use but also in relation to heavy maternal alcohol and drug use in pregnancy and, in many countries, the overall pattern of HIV spread. The second point is that, while a considerable amount of such 'problem behaviour' is linked with social disadvantage, it is not confined to such disadvantage.

Most of the evidence considered in this book relates to Britain or the USA. It is evident that there are differences between these two countries. It is equally certain that further differences would emerge from studies of youth risks elsewhere, especially in developing countries. Patterns of risk-taking are strongly influenced by social and cultural factors. The latter inevitably mean that levels of association and the predictive relationships between different types of risk will vary markedly between different societies. Accordingly, caution is required when attempting to generalize on the basis of data collection in a single location.

The complex aetiology of psychoactive drug use imposes major constraints upon action designed to curb drug misuse. Similar problems beset attempts to modify sexual behaviour or other forms of risk-taking. People, particularly young people, are not rational, but often view themselves as exceptional and invulnerable. Some have such low self-esteem and few aspirations that 'risk' is simply an alien concept.

It has been stated repeatedly in the text of this book that risk-taking is influenced by complex factors. This can be illustrated with reference to two forms of behaviour, vehicle driving and sexual behaviour.

Driving may involve risk at a number of different levels. On one level are badly repaired roads, poor road or warning signs or defective traffic lights; at another level are poor weather conditions. The more personally controllable level for the driver includes speeding, unsafe overtaking, driving too close to other vehicles, failure to wear seat belts, poor vehicle maintenance and the consumption of alcohol or other drugs. Other problems include the proximity of other speeding and/or intoxicated or careless drivers, or pedestrians. Peer pressures may encourage young drivers and their passengers to travel too fast or to consume intoxicating quantities of alcohol, illicit or prescribed drugs. Under many situations a cumulative process of risk may occur in which alcohol or other drugs interact with a variety of other factors any of which in isolation would constitute a lesser degree of hazard. A sober driver can negotiate a busy road far better than an intoxicated driver, encouraged by drunken friends.

Sexual encounters may provide quite different risk situations. The initiation of such an encounter typically involves a number of steps. Initial dating often involves both insecurity, uncertainty and the consumption of alcohol or illicit drugs. A series of verbal and other cues are involved in an explicit or implicit agreement to engage in some form of sexual activity. The issue of condom use is often perceived as highly problematic. It may signify a change in the relationship, by introducing a 'clinical' aspect into a highly emotional situation. Condom use also introduces a note of rational responsibility into a previously instinctive and non-logical relationship. Condom use may be daunting for inexperienced males. It is likely to be far more so for young females. The latter may be inhibited for a variety of reasons. Females have to request or negotiate condom use in a way that is often alien to both partners' perceptions of sex roles.

These two examples simply provide an indication of some of the factors and processes that are often involved in risk-taking. In particular, it is noted that to refrain from certain risks may necessitate resisting overwhelming social pressures or strong emotions and drives. Risks are often taken in association with others who provide encouragement and who may actively deter risk avoidance or the adoption of harm minimization procedures. The latter may be derided as 'wimpish' or cowardly. Under such circumstances nobody is present to point out the existence or magnitude of a risk.

Males generally drink more and use illicit drugs more than females. Individuals may be inclined to drink or use other drugs more rapidly in an all-male group than in a mixed sex group. This may lead to sudden high levels of alcohol or drugs in the blood stream. Such situations are likely to engender higher levels of risk-taking. Even so the precise relationship between alcohol and other drug use and risk-taking remains unclear. The effects of a drug involve an interaction between the individual, the drug and the social setting. 'Disinhibition' probably involves an interaction between the chemistry or dose of a drug and beliefs and misconceptions about the supposed effects to be expected or desired. There are sex differences in drug effects and the latter are certainly strongly influenced by a host of social and cultural factors.

Orford (1985) has noted that people may have 'excessive appetites' for a number of things, which, though not drugs, may involve a dependence-like attachment. The internal chemistry of the human brain remains ill charted as yet. It is known that the brain secretes substances similar to depressant and stimulant drugs. It is possible that sexual arousal, due to the substances this triggers in the brain, has much in common with some of the pleasant sensations derived from drug use. Such chemical effects interact with the personality, social and cultural mores of those involved to form a potent set of drives and responses.

As indicated in the preceding chapter, the aim of much health education is risk reduction. Such 'successes' raise an important possibility, namely that a reduction in one type of risk may be accompanied by the adoption of alternative risks. As indicated in Chapter 3, there has been a substantial decline in tobacco use during recent years. Is this somehow connected to the steady rise in illicit drug use, or the establishment of a relatively stable and chronic level of alcohol misuse?

A huge literature already exists in relation to the youthful use of legal and illicit drugs and evidence related to sexual behaviour has been generated by concern about AIDS. In spite of this, 'risk' remains a mysterious topic. Much remains to be discovered about the interacting processes that contribute to risk. Health education, or strategies to curb or minimize certain risk-taking behaviours, is seriously impeded by this lack of basic knowledge. At the same time it is illogical for one risk, such as drug injection, to be wholly condemned while others, such as cave exploration or hang-gliding, are esteemed.

The endemic nature of the drive to take risks and the multiple and powerful forces which foster such behaviours present an overriding reality. Moreover, some of the most extreme and dangerous behaviours are associated with major chronic inequalities in health and social resources. These immense considerations render attempts to 'stamp out' risk-taking forlorn and ineffective. Risk elimination, though in some areas desirable, is, in relation to many of the topics considered in this book, simply unattainable. This is because the complete elimination of risks would necessitate removing all of the inequalities in social and life opportunities (good) as well as changing human nature (not necessarily so good). 'Just Say No' is a vacuous, silly slogan.

In spite of the major constraints that do limit scope for social and health policy a number of positive conclusions are justified. The first is that risk-related behaviour can be influenced. The move away from cigarette smoking and the equally impressive fall in alcohol-involved road deaths in the United Kingdom provide important examples of youthful behaviour change in the right direction. Illicit drug use by young people in the USA has also recently declined. Health education should not be confused with high profile, politicized campaigning. Health education is, however, well worth pursuing and there is probably a greater awareness than ever before of the need for such education to be experimental and properly assessed. All of the health risks referred to in preceding pages are worthy targets for public policy. At present the authors conclude that harm minimization is a far more realistic approach than grandiose activities which simply exhort, or seek to denigrate particular behaviour for unspecified or possibly unjustified reasons. Factual accuracy is important. Heroin does not necessarily screw you up. People do not necessarily die of ignorance.

AIDS has emerged during the past decade as by far the greatest potential health threat to the young. Traditional responses to health issues and to other public policy considerations need to be urgently revised in order to curb the spread of the AIDS epidemic.

AIDS IS A FAR GREATER PUBLIC HEALTH THREAT THAN EVEN THE MISUSE OF TOBACCO, ALCOHOL, ILLICIT AND PRESCRIBED DRUGS

Most of those who use or even misuse psychoactives drugs do not die prematurely thereby. AIDS, in contrast, spares nobody.

The arrival of HIV infection and AIDS now necessitates the adoption of vigorous proactive public health measures aimed primarily, but by no means exclusively, at the sexually active and drug-using young. Gratifying, but so far purely limited, success has been achieved by a variety of approaches, some of which were noted in the previous chapter. Traditional policies towards illicit drug use and prostitution must be reconsidered to ensure that they do not contribute to the spread of AIDS: even so, some police officers continue to use possession of condoms as evidence of illicit street prostitution or of brothel keeping. Such policies are now dangerous to the health of the whole community. Many traditional prejudices constitute enormous obstacles to AIDS prevention.

It should be noted that there is a crucial difference between an individual's risk from a specific behaviour and the overall social level of risks associated with the same behaviour. The concept of the 'Preventive Paradox' was originally described in relation to cardiovascular disease by Rose (1981). This has been applied to the topic of alcohol misuse by Kreitman (1986). In brief, this paradox draws attention to the fact that the greatest level of risk is experienced by those who are the most 'extreme' cases, such as the heaviest drinkers or drug users. Such individuals place themselves at a high level of *personal risk*. However, such people are rare. The greatest impact on the *overall social level* of harm, such as alcohol misuse, will be achieved, not by influencing the 'extreme' minority, but by influencing the less extreme majority. As Kreitman has commented:

> reducing the likelihood of harm for a group of individuals has been erroneously equated with the optimum strategy for reducing the likelihood of harm for the population at large. While both types of reduction are desirable they are not equivalent.
>
> (Kreitman 1986: 354)

This perspective is convincing. It immediately confronts two major practical problems. The first is that the 'extreme' individuals may be difficult to detect, contact and influence. The second is that people whose behaviours are not 'extreme' are likely to be highly resistant to the notion that they have any need to change them. These facts present major problems for both public policy and for the implementation of preventive strategies.

More research is needed to illuminate the patterns and inter-relationships of risky behaviours, both at specific points of time and over extended periods, up to and including the life course. In addition, current research evidence is largely based upon small ad hoc studies. More prospective research is needed to monitor changing behaviours over time.

Nobody is going to prevent young men and women from taking risks. Even so, it is obvious that the scale of such risks can be influenced for the better. During recent years rock climbers have greatly reduced their risks thanks to the introduction of better ropes, boots, helmets and other equipment. Climbing remains as exciting as ever since enthusiasts have been able to balance their new technology by climbing far more difficult grades of route. The analogy between this particular brand of risk-taking and some of the other activities cited in this book should not be pressed too far. There are, however, obvious parallels between one type of risk and others.

In conclusion, it should be acknowledged that the majority of people do not drink, smoke, use drugs or have sexual intercourse because they want to harm themselves or others. Most adolescents simply enjoy these things. They are no different from others in this respect. Moreover, 'young people' are not a separate species, even though they often appear to their elders as a separate tribe. Their risks are also society's risks. Very often their behaviours reflect, even imitate, those of their parents and of others from their social backgrounds. It is not helpful to scapegoat young people as the demons responsible for today's health problems. Most of us are drug users in a drug-using world. Our problem is to reconcile the things we enjoy with the damage these pleasures can inflict.

Bibliography

This bibliography lists the references which were useful in writing this book. Not all were cited directly in the text.

Aaro, L.E., Bruland, E., Hauknes, A. and Lochsen, P.M. (1983). 'Smoking among Norwegian school children 1975–1980, III, The effect of anti-smoking campaigns', *Scandinavian Journal of Psychology*, 24, 1–7.

Abel, E.L. and Sokol, R.J. (1986). 'Fetal alcohol syndrome is now leading cause of mental retardation', *Lancet*, II, 1222.

Abel, E.L. and Sokol, R.J. (1987). 'Incidence of fetal alcohol syndrome and economic impact of FAS-related anomalies', *Drug and Alcohol Dependence*, 19, 51–70.

Adler, N.E., Kegeles, S.M., Irwin, C.E. and Wibblesman, C. (1990). 'Adolescent contraceptive behavior: an assessment of decision process', *Journal of Pediatrics*, 110, 463–71.

Advisory Council on the Misuse of Drugs (1982). *Treatment and Rehabilitation*, London, Department of Health and Social Security.

Advisory Council on the Misuse of Drugs (1984). *Prevention*, London, Home Office.

Advisory Council on the Misuse of Drugs (1988). *AIDS and Drug Misuse, Part 1*, London, HMSO.

Advisory Council on the Misuse of Drugs (1989). *AIDS and Drug Misuse, Part 2*, London, HMSO.

Aggleton, P. (1987). *Deviance*, London, Tavistock.

Aitken, P.P. (1978). *Ten-to-Fourteen Year Olds and Alcohol*, Edinburgh, HMSO.

Aitken, P.P. and Leathar, D.S. (1981). *Adults' Attitudes Towards Drinking and Smoking Among Young People in Scotland*, Vol. IV, Edinburgh, HMSO.

Amaro, H., Fried, L.E., Cabral, H. and Zuckerman, B. (1990). 'Violence during programmes and substance abuse', *American Journal of Public Health*, 80, 575–9.

Anderson, D.O. and Ferris, B.G. (1962). 'Role of tobacco smoking in the causation of chronic respiratory disease', *New England Journal of Medicine*, 267, 787–94.

Anderson, P. (1991). *Management of Drinking Problems*, Copenhagen, World Health Organization.

Answer (1990a). *AIDS News Supplement Weekly Report*, Glasgow, Communicable Diseases (Scotland) Unit, Ruchill Hospital (CDS90/33).

Answer (1990b). *AIDS News Supplement Weekly Report*, Glasgow, Communicable Diseases (Scotland) Unit, Ruchill Hospital (CDS90/51–2).

Answer (1991a). *AIDS News Supplement Weekly Report*, Glasgow, Communicable Diseases (Scotland) Unit, Ruchill Hospital (CDS91/04).

Answer (1991b). *AIDS News Supplement Weekly Report*, Glasgow, Communicable Diseases (Scotland) Unit, Ruchill Hospital (CDS91/05).

Aral, S.O. and Cates, W. (1989). 'The multiple dimensions of sexual behaviour as risk factor for sexually transmitted disease: the sexually experienced are not necessarily more active', *Sexually Transmitted Diseases*, 16, 173–7.

Armytage, W.H.G., Chester, R. and Peel, J. (1980). *Changing Patterns of Sexual Behaviour*, London, Academic Press.

Bachrach, C.A. and Horn, M.C. (1988). 'Sexual activity among US women of reproductive age', *American Journal of Public Health*, 78, 320–1.

Bagnall, G. (1988). 'Use of alcohol, tobacco and illicit drugs amongst 13-year-olds in three areas of Britain', *Drug and Alcohol Dependence*, 22, 241–51.

Bagnall, G. (1991a). 'Alcohol and drug use in a Scottish cohort: 10 years on', *British Journal of Addiction*, 86, 895–904.

Bagnall, G. (1991b). Personal communication.

Bagnall, G. (1991c). *Educating Young Drinkers*, London, Tavistock/Routledge.

Bagnall, G. (1991d). 'Survey research and HIV-related behaviours: a case for caution', *Health Education Journal*, 50, 171–3.

Bagnall, G., Plant, M.A. and Warwick, W. (1990). 'Alcohol, drugs and AIDS-related risks: results from a prospective study', *AIDS Care*, 2, 309–17.

Bagnall, G. and Plant, M.A. (1991). 'AIDS risks, alcohol and illicit drug use amongst young adults in areas of high and low rates of HIV infection', *AIDS Care*, 3, 355–61.

Bakalar, J.B. and Grinspoon, L. (1984). *Drug Control in a Free Society*, Cambridge, Cambridge University Press.

Balassone, M.L. (1989). 'Risk of contraceptive discontinuation among adolescents', *Journal of Adolescent Health Care*, 10, 527–33.

Bancroft, J. (1983). *Human Sexuality and Its Problems*, Edinburgh, Churchill Livingstone.

Bandura, A. (1984). '"Self-efficacy". Toward a unifying theory of behavioral change', *Psychology Review*, 84, 191–215.

Bandy, P. and President, P.A. (1983). 'Recent literature on drug abuse and prevention and mass media: focussing on youth, parents, women and the elderly', *Journal of Drug Education*, 13, 255–71.

Barnard, M. and McKeganey, N. (1990). 'Adolescents, sex and injecting drug use: risks for HIV infection', *AIDS Care* 2, 103–16.

Barnes, G.G. and Noble, P. (1972). 'Deprivation and drug addiction – a study of a vulnerable sub-group', *British Journal of Social Work*, 2, 299–311.

Bauer, J. (1982). *Alcoholism and Women*, Toronto, Inner City Books.

Baumrind, D. (1987). 'A developmental perspective on adolescent risk taking in contemporary America'. In: Irwin, C.E. jnr. (ed.) *Adolescent Social Behavior and Health*, San Francisco, Jossey Bass, pp. 93–125.

Beattie, J.O., Day, F.E., Cockburn, F. and Garg, R.A. (1983). 'Alcohol and the foetus in the West of Scotland', *British Medical Journal*, 287, 17–20.

Beattie, M. (1987). *Codependent No More*, Minnesota, Hazelden.

Bell, C.G. and Battjes, R. (eds) (1985). *Prevention Research: Deterring Drug*

Abuse Among Children and Adolescents, Rockville, Maryland, National Institute on Drug Abuse.

Bennet, G. (ed.) (1989). *Treating Drug Abusers*, London, Tavistock/Routledge.

Berridge, V. and Edwards, G. (1981). *Opium and the People*, London, Allen Lane.

Bevan, N. (1988). *AIDS and Drugs*, London, Gloucester Press.

Bewley, B.R. and Bland, J.M. (1976). 'Smoking and respiratory symptoms in two groups of school children', *Preventive Medicine*, 5, 63–9.

Bewley, B.R. and Bland, J.M. (1978). 'The child's image of a young smoker', *Health Education*, 37, 236–41.

Biglan, A., Metzler, C.W., Wirt, R., Ary, D., Noell, J., Ochs, L., French, C. and Hood, D. (1990). 'Social and behavioral factors associated with high risk sexual behavior among adolescents', *Journal of Behavioral Medicine*, 13, 245–61.

Binnie, H.L. and Murdock, G. (1969). 'The attitudes to drugs and drug takers of students of the university and colleges of higher education in an English Midland city', University of Leicester, *Vaughan Papers*, 14, 1–29.

Bland, J.M., Bewley, B.R., Pollard, V. and Banks, M.H. (1978). 'Effects of children's and parent's smoking on respiratory systems', *Archives of the Disturbed Child*, 53, 100–5.

Blumberg, H.H. (1981). 'Characteristics of people coming into treatment'. In: Edwards, G. and Busch, C. (eds) *Drug Problems in Britain*, London, Academic Press, pp. 77–116.

Bonington, C.J. (1981). *Quest for Adventure*, London, Hodder & Stoughton.

Bostock, Y. and Davies, J.K. (1979). 'Recent changes in the prevalence of cigarette smoking in Scotland', *Health Bulletin*, 37, 260–7.

Bowie, C. and Ford, N. (1989). 'Sexual behaviour of young people and the risk of HIV infection', *Journal of Epidemiology and Community Health*, 43, 61–5.

Box, S. (1987). *Recession, Crime and Punishment*, London, Macmillan.

Brain, P.F. (ed.) (1986). *Alcohol and Aggression*. London, Croom Helm.

Breeze, E. (1985a). *Women and Drinking*, London, HMSO.

Breeze, E. (1985b). *Differences in Drinking Patterns Between Selected Regions*, London, HMSO.

Brenner, J., Hernando-Briongos P. and Goos, C. (1991). *AIDS Among Drug Abusers in Europe*, Copenhagen, World Health Organization.

Brewers' Society (1990). *Statistical Handbook*, London, Brewers' Society.

British Medical Association (1986). *Young People and Alcohol*, London, British Medical Association.

British Medical Journal (1985). 'Media drugs campaigns may be worse than a waste of money' (leading article), *British Medical Journal*, 290, 416.

Brown, C. and Lawton, J. (1988). *Illicit Drug Use in Portsmouth and Havant*, London, Policy Studies Institute.

Bruun, K., Edwards, G., Lumio, M., Makela, K., Osterberg, E., Pan, L., Popham, R.E., Room, R., Schmidt, W., Skog, O-J. and Sulkenen, P. (1975). *Alcohol Control Policies in Public Health Perspective*, Helsinki, Finnish Foundation for Alcohol Studies.

Bruun, K., Pan, L. and Rexed, I. (1979). *The Gentlemen's Club: International Control of Drugs and Alcohol*, Chicago, Chicago University Press.

Bucknall, A.B.V. and Robertson, J.R. (1986). 'Deaths of heroin users in a general practice', *Journal of the Royal College of General Practitioners*, 36, 120–2.

Burroughs, W. (1959). *The Naked Lunch*, Paris, Olympia.

Callari, S. and Mikus, R. (1990). 'Correlates of adolescent sexual behavior', *Psychological Reports*, 66, 1179–84.

Cavan, S. (1966). *Liquor License: An Ethnography of Bar Behavior*, Chicago, Aldine.

Central Policy Review Staff (1979). *Alcohol Policies in the United Kingdom*, Stockholm, Sociologiska Institutionen, Stockholms Universitat.

Chambers, G. and Tombs, J. (eds) (1984). *The British Crime Survey, Scotland, A Scottish Research Study*. Edinburgh, HMSO.

Chasnoff, I.J. (ed.) (1986). *Drug Use in Pregnancy*, Boston, MTP Press Ltd.

Chatlos, C. (1987). *Crack*, New York, Lawrence Chilnick.

Christiaens, L. (1961). 'La descendance des alcooliques' (The offspring of alcoholics), *American Pediatrics*, 37, 380.

Christiaens, L., Mizon, J.P. and Delmarle, G. (1960). 'Sur la descendance des alcooliques' (On the offspring of alcoholics), *American Pediatrics*, 36, 37.

Clarke, J., Abram, R. and Monteiro, E.F. (1990). 'The sexual behaviour and knowledge about AIDS in a group of adolescent girls in Leeds', *Genitourinary Medicine*, 66, 189–92.

Cliff, K.S., Grout, P. and Machin, D. (1982). 'Smoking and attitudes to seat belt usage', *Public Health*, 96, 48–52.

Coffey, T.G. (1966). 'Beer Street, Gin Lane: some views of 18th century drinking'. *Quarterly Journal of Studies on Alcohol*, 27, 690–2.

Coggans, N., Shewan, D., Henderson, M., Davies, J.B. and O'Hagan, F. (1989). *National Evaluation of Drug Education in Scotland*, Centre for Occupational and Health Psychology, University of Strathclyde.

Cohen, S. (1972). *Folk Devils and Moral Panics*, London, Granada.

Collins, J.J. jnr (1982). *Drinking and Crime*, London, Tavistock.

Collins, S. (ed.) (1990). *Alcohol, Social Work and Helping*, London, Tavistock/ Routledge.

Commission of the European Communities (1986). *Statistics of Smoking in the Member States of the European Community*, Luxembourg, Office for Official Publications of the European Communities.

Concise Oxford Dictionary (1983), Oxford, Clarendon Press.

Co-operative Wholesale Society (1991). *Anti-Social – Who Cares?* London, Co-operative Wholesale Society Ltd.

Corder, B.W., Smith, R.A. and Swisher, J.D. (1975). *Drug Abuse Prevention*, Dubuque, Iowe, Wm. C. Brown.

Courtwright, D.T. (1982). *Dark Paradise*, Cambridge, Massachusetts, Harvard University Press.

Crawford, A., Plant, M.A., Kreitman, N. and Latcham, R. (1984). 'Regional variations in alcohol-related morbidity in Britain: a myth uncovered? II. Population survey', *British Medical Journal*, 289, 1343–9.

Curran, J.W., Jaffe, H.W., Hardy, A.M., Morgan, W.M., Selick, R.M. and Dondero, T.J. (1989). 'Epidemiology of AIDS and HIV infection in the United States'. In: Kulstad, R. (ed.) *AIDS 1988*, Washington, DC, American Association for the Advancement of Science, pp. 19–34.

Curtis, H.A., Lawrence, C.J. and Tripp, J.H. (1988). 'Teenage sexual intercourse and pregnancy', *Archives of Disease in Childhood*, 63, 373–9.

Davidson, R., Rollnick, S. and MacEwan, I. (eds) (1991). *Counselling Problem Drinkers*, London, Tavistock/Routledge.

Davies, J.B. (1991). Personal communication.

Davies, J.B. and Stacey, B. (1972). *Teenagers and Alcohol: A developmental study in Glasgow*, London, HMSO.

Davies, P.T. and Walsh, D. (1983). *Alcohol Problems and Alcohol Control Policies in Europe*, London, Croom Helm.

Dehaene, P.H., Crepin, G., Walbaum, R., Titran, M., Samaille-Villette, D.H. and Somaille, P. (1977). 'La descendance des mères alcooliques chroniques: à propos de 16 cas d'alcoolisme foetal' (Offspring of chronic alcoholic mothers: a report of 16 cases), *Revue Français de Gynécologie et d'Obstétrique*, 72, 492.

Department of Health and Social Security/Welsh Office (1987). *AIDS: Monitoring Responses to the Public Education Campaign February 1986–February 1987*, London, HMSO.

Department of Health (1991). Personal communication.

Department of Transport (1990a). *Road Accidents Great Britain: The Casualty Report*, Government Statistical Office.

Department of Transport (1990b). *Blood Alcohol Levels in Fatalities in Great Britain 1988*, Transport and Road Research Laboratory.

Des Jarlais, D.G. and Friedman, S.R. (1988). 'HIV infection and intravenous drug use', *AIDS*, 2, 5–6.

Dight, S. (1976). *Scottish Drinking Habits*, London, HMSO.

Dobbs, J. and Marsh, A. (1983). *Smoking Among Secondary School Children*, London, HMSO.

Dobbs, J. and Marsh, A. (1985). *Smoking Among Secondary School Children in 1984*, London, HMSO.

Doll, R. and Hill, A.B. (1952). 'A study of the aetiology of carcinoma of the lung', *British Medical Journal*, 2, 1271–6.

Doll, R. and Hill, A.B. (1964). 'Mortality in relation to smoking: ten years' observation of British doctors', *British Medical Journal*, 1, 1399–410, 1460–7.

Doll, R. and Peto, R. (1986). 'Mortality in relation to smoking: 20 years observation on male British doctors', *British Medical Journal*, ii, 1525–36.

Donoghoe, M.C. (1991). 'Syringe exchange: has it worked?' *Druglink*, January–February, 8–11.

Donoghoe, M.C., Stimson, G.V. and Dolan, K. (1989). 'Sexual behaviour of injecting drug users and associated risks of HIV infection for non-injecting sexual partners', *AIDS Care*, 1, 51–8.

Donoghoe, M.C., Stimson, G.V., Dolan, K. and Alldritt, L. (1989). 'Changes in risk behaviour in clients of syringe-exchange schemes in England and Scotland', *AIDS*, 3, 267–72.

Donovan, C. (1990). 'Adolescent sexuality', *British Medical Journal*, 30, 1026–7.

Donovan, J.E. and Jessor, R. (1978). 'Adolescent problem drinking: psychosocial correlates in a national sample study', *Journal of Studies on Alcohol*, 39, 1506–24.

Donovan, J.E. and Jessor, R. (1985). 'Structure of problem behavior in adolescence and young adulthood', *Journal of Consulting and Clinical Psychology*, 53, 890–904.

Donovan, J.E., Jessor, R. and Costa, R. (1988). 'The syndrome of problem behavior in adolescence: a replication', *Journal of Consulting and Clinical Psychology*, 56, 762–5.

Dorn, N. (1981). 'Social analyses of drugs in health education and the media'. In: Edwards, G. and Busch, C. (eds) *Drug Problems in Britain*, London, Academic Press, pp. 281–304.

Dorn, N. and South, N. (1983). *Message in a Bottle*, London, Gower.

Dorn, N. and South, N. (1987). *A Land Fit for Heroin?*, London, Macmillan.

Dorris, M. (1989). *The Broken Cord*, New York, Harper & Row.

Dowling, J. and Maclennan, A. (1978). *The Chemically Dependent Woman*, Toronto, Addiction Research Foundation.

Duffy, J.C. (1991). *Trends in Alcohol Consumption Patterns 1978–1989*, Henley on Thames, NTC Publications.

Dunbar, J.A. (1985). *A Quiet Massacre*, London, Institute of Alcohol Studies, Occasional Paper no. 7.

Du Rant, R.H. and Saunders, J.M. (1989). 'Sexual behavior and contraceptive risk taking among sexually active females', *Journal of Adolescent Health Care*, 10, 1–9.

Durex (1990a). *The Durex Report*, London, LRC Products Ltd.

Durex (1990b). *AIDS Newsletter*, London, LRC Products Ltd.

Edwards, G. (1991). *Addictions: Personal Influences and Scientific Movement*, New Brunswick, Transaction.

Edwards, G. and Raw, M. (1991). 'The tobacco habit as drug dependence', *British Journal of Addiction*, 86, 483–4.

Einstein, R. (1975). 'Patterns of use of alcohol, cannabis and tobacco in a student population', *British Journal of Addiction*, 70, 145–50.

Eiser, J.R., Sutton, S.R. and Wober, M. (1979). 'Smoking, seat belts, and beliefs about health', *Addictive Behaviors*, 4, 331–8.

Elkind, D. (1967). 'Egocentrism in adolescence', *Child Development*, 30, 1025–34.

Elkind, D. (1984). 'Teenage thinking: implications for health care', *Pediatric Nursing*, 10, 383–5.

Elkind, D. (1985). 'Cognitive development and adolescent disabilities', *Journal of Adolescent Health Care*, 6, 84–9.

Elkington, J. (1986). *The Poisoned Womb*, Harmondsworth, Pelican.

Evans, L., Wasielewski, P. and von Buseck, C.R. (1982). 'Compulsory seat belt usage and driver risk-taking behavior', *Human Factors*, 24, 41–8.

Fagin, L. and Little, M. (1984). *The Forsaken Families*, Harmondsworth, Penguin.

Farrell, C. (1978). *My Mother Said: The Way Young People Learned About Sex and Birth Control*, London, Routledge & Kegan Paul.

Fay, R.E., Turner, C.F., Klassen, A.D. and Gagnon, J.H. (1989). 'Prevalence and patterns of some gender sexual contact among men', *Science*, 243, 338–48.

Fazey, C. (1977). *The Aetiology of Psychoactive Substance Use*, Paris, Unesco.

Fee, E. and Fox, D.M. (eds) (1988). *AIDS: The Burden of History*, Berkeley, University of California Press.

Feldstein, J.H. and Washburn, D.E. (1980). 'Shifts toward risk in adults at three age levels', *Experimental Ageing Research*, 6, 149–57.

Fillmore, K.M. (1988). *Alcohol Use across the Life Course*, Toronto, Addiction Research Foundation.

Fingarette, H. (1988). *Heavy Drinking: The Myth of Alcoholism as a Disease*, Berkeley, University of California Press.

Finnegan, L.P. (1982). 'Outcome of children born to women dependent upon narcotics'. In: Stimmel, B. (ed.) *The Effects of Maternal Alcohol and Drug Abuse on the Newborn*, New York, Haworth.

Fish, F., Wells, B., Bindeman, G., Bunney, J. and Jordan, M. (1974). 'Prevalence of drug misuse amongst young people in Glasgow 1970–1972'. *British Journal of Addiction*, 69, 231–6.

Fishbein, M. and Ajzen, I. (1975). *Belief, Attitude, Intention and Behavior: An Introduction to Theory and Research*, Massachusetts, Addison-Wesley.

Flanigan, B. and Hitch, M. (1986). 'Alcohol use and sexual intercourse and contraception: an exploratory study', *Journal of Alcohol and Drug Education*, 31, 6–40.
Flanigan, B., McLean, A., Hall, C. and Propp, V. (1990). 'Alcohol use as a situational influence on young women's pregnancy risk-taking behaviors', *Adolescence*, xxv, 97, 205–14.
Ford, N. (1989). 'Urban–rural variations in the level of heterosexual activity of young people', *Area*, 21, 237–48.
Ford, N. (1990a). *Psycho-Active Drug Use, Sexual Activity and AIDS Awareness of Young People in Bristol*, Institute of Population Studies, University of Exeter.
Ford, N. (1990b). *AIDS Awareness and Socio-Sexual Lifestyles of Young People in Exeter and District*, Exeter, Institute of Population Studies, University of Exeter.
Foreman, D. and Chilvers, C. (1989). 'Sexual behaviour of young and middle aged men in England and Wales', *British Medical Journal*, 298, 1137–42.
Forrest, F., du V Florey, C., McPherson, F. and Young, J.A. (1991). 'Reported social alcohol consumption during pregnancy and infants' development at 18 months', *British Medical Journal*, 303, 22–6.
Fossey, E. (1992). Personal communication.
Foster, K., Wilmot, A. and Dobbs, J. (1990). *General Household Survey 1988*, London, HMSO.
Frank, D.I. and Lang, A.R. (1990). 'Alcohol use and sexual arousal research: application of the health belief model', *Nurse Practitioner*, 15, 32–5.
Freemantle, B. (1985). *The Fix*, London, Corgi.
Friedman, K.M. (1975). *Public Policies and the Smoking Health Controversy*, Lexington, Lexington Books.
Frogatt, P. (1988). *Smoking and Health*, Further Report of the Independent Scientific Committee, London, HMSO.
Fullilove, R.E., Fullilove, H.T., Bowser, B. and Gross, S. (1990). 'Crack users: the new AIDS risk group?', *Cancer Detection and Prevention*, 14, 363–8.
Galt, M., Gillies, P.A. and Wilson, K. (1989). 'Surveying knowledge and attitudes towards AIDS in young adults – just 19', *Health Education Journal*, 48, 162–6.
Ghodse, H., Sheehay, M., Taylor, C. and Edwards, G. (1985). 'Deaths of drug addicts in the United Kingdom 1962–1981', *British Medical Journal*, 290, 429–38.
Ghodsian, M. and Power, C. (1987). 'Alcohol consumption between the ages of 16 and 23 in Britain: a longitudinal study', *British Journal of Addiction*, 82, 175–80.
Gibson, G.T., Baghurst, P.A. and Colley, D.P. (1983). 'Maternal alcohol, tobacco and cannabis consumption and the outcome of pregnancy', *Australia and New Zealand Journal of Obstetrics and Gynaecology*, 23, 15–19.
Giesbrecht, N., Gonzalez, R., Grant, M., Osterberg, E., Room, R., Rootman, I. and Towle, L. (eds) (1989). *Drinking and Casualties: Accidents, Poisonings and Violence in an International Perspective*. London, Tavistock/Routledge.
Gillies, P.A. (1989). 'A longitudinal study of hopes and worries of adolescents', *Journal of Adolescence*, 12, 69–81.
Gillies, P.A. (1991). 'HIV infection, alcohol and illicit drugs', *Current Opinion in Psychiatry*, 4, 448–53.
Gillies, P.A. and Carballo, M. (1990). 'Adult perception of risk, risk behaviour and HIV/AIDS: a focus for intervention and research', *AIDS*, 4, 943–51.
Gillies, P.A., Madeley, R.J. and Power, F.L. (1989). 'Why do pregnant women smoke?', *Public Health*, 103, 337–44.
Gillies, P., Pearson, J.C.G. and Elwood, J.M. (1986). 'Survey of smoking in 15–16 year olds', Department of Community Health, University of Nottingham.

Gillies, P. and Willcox, B. (1984). 'Reducing the risk of smoking amongst the young', *Public Health*, 98, 49–54.

Glaser, D. and Snow, M. (1969). *Public Knowledge and Attitudes to Drug Use*, New York, Addiction Control Commission.

Glassner, B. and Loughlin, J. (1987). *Drugs in Adolescents' Worlds*, London, Macmillan.

Goddard, E. (1989). *Smoking among Secondary School Children in England in 1988*, London, HMSO.

Goddard, E. (1990). *Why Children Start Smoking*, London, HMSO.

Goddard, E. (1991). *Drinking in England and Wales in the Late 1980s*, London, HMSO.

Goddard, E. and Ikin, C. (1987). *Smoking among Secondary School Children in 1986*, London, HMSO.

Goddard, E. and Ikin, C. (1988). *Drinking in England and Wales in 1987*, London, HMSO.

Godfrey, C. and Robinson, D. (eds) (1990). *Preventing Alcohol and Tobacco Problems*, Vol. 2, Aldershot, Avebury.

Goetz, D., Hall, S., Harbison, R. and Reid, M. (1988). 'Pediatric acquired immuno-deficiency syndrome with negative human immunodeficiency virus by enzyme-linked immunoabsorbent assay and western blot', *Paediatrics*, 81, 356–9.

Goldbaum, G.M., Remington, P.L., Powell, K.E., Hogelin, G. and Gentry, E.M., (1986). 'Failure to use seat belts in the United States, *Journal of the American Medical Association*, 255, 2459–62.

Goode, E. (1970). *The Marihuana Smokers*, New York, Basic Books.

Goode, E. (1972). *Drugs in American Society*, New York, Knopf.

Goodwin, D. (1976). *Is Alcoholism Hereditary?*, New York, Oxford University Press.

Gossop, M. (1987). *Living with Drugs*, London, Wildwood House.

Grant, L.M. and Demetriou, E. (1988). 'Adolescent sexuality', *The Pediatric Clinics of North America*, 35, 1271–89.

Grant, M. (ed.) (1985). *Alcohol Policies*, Copenhagen, World Health Organization.

Grant, M., Plant, M.A. and Williams, A. (eds) (1983). *Economics and Alcohol*, London, Croom Helm.

Grant, M. and Ritson, E.B. (eds) (1983). *Alcohol: The Prevention Debate*, London, Croom Helm.

Green, G., MacIntyre, S., West, P. and Ecob, R. (1991). 'Like parent like child? Associations between drinking and smoking behaviour of parents and their children', *British Journal of Addiction*, 86, 745–58.

Greenwood, J. (1990). 'Creating a new drug service in Edinburgh', *British Medical Journal*, 300, 587–9.

Greydanus, D.E. (1987). 'Risk-taking behaviors in adolescence', *Journal of the American Medical Association*, 258, 2110.

Grout, P., Cliff, K.S., Harman, M.L. and Machin, D. (1983). 'Cigarette smoking, road traffic accidents and seat belt usage', *Public Health*, 97, 95–101.

Haavio-Mannila, E. (ed.) (1989). *Women, Alcohol and Drugs in the Nordic Countries*, Helsinki, Nordic Council for Alcohol and Drug Research.

Haggard, H.W. and Jellinek, E.M. (1942). *Alcohol Explored*, New York, Doubleday.

Halliday, H.L., Reid, M.M.L. and McClure, G. (1982) 'Results of heavy drinking in pregnancy', *British Journal of Obstetrics and Gynaecology*, 89, 892–5.

Halmesmaki, E., Raivio, K.O. and Ylikorkala, O. (1987). 'Patterns of alcohol consumption during pregnancy', *Obstetrics and Gynaecology*, 69, 594–7.

Harlap, S. and Shiona, P.H. (1980). 'Alcohol, smoking and the incidence of spontaneous abortion in the first and second trimester', *Lancet*, II, 173–6.

Harpwood, D. (1981). *Tea and Tranquillisers*, London, Virago.

Hartnoll, R., Lewis, R., Mitcheson, M. and Bryer, S. (1985). 'Estimating the prevalence of opioid dependence', *The Lancet*, I, 26 January, 203–5.

Havard, J. (1986). 'Drunken driving among the young', *British Medical Journal*, 293, 774.

Hawker, A. (1978). *Adolescents and Alcohol*, London, Edsall.

Hayder, M.R. and Nelson, M.M. (1978). 'The foetal alcohol syndrome', *South African Medical Journal*, 54, 571.

Health Education Authority (1989). *Young People's Health and Lifestyles Survey (9–15 year olds)*, London, MORI.

Health Education Authority (1990). *Young People's Health and Lifestyles Survey (16–19 year olds)*, London, MORI.

Heather, N. and Robertson, I. (1981). *Controlled Drinking*, London, Methuen.

Heather, N. and Robertson, I. (1986). *Problem Drinking*, Harmondsworth, Pelican.

Henman, A., Lewis, R. and Malyon, T. (1985). *Big Deal: The Politics of the Illicit Drugs Business*, London, Pluto.

Henningfield, J.E., Cohen, C. and Slade, J.D. (1991). 'Is nicotine more addictive than cocaine?', *British Journal of Addiction*, 86, 565–9.

Hingson, R. (1983). 'FAS-like symptoms seen in pot-smokers newborn?', *The Journal*, 1 January, 2, Toronto, Addiction Research Foundation.

Hingson, R., Albert, J.J., Day, N., Dooling, E., Kayne, H., Morelock, S., Oppenheimer, E. and Zuckerman, B. (1982). 'Effects of maternal drinking and marijuana use on fetal growth and development', *Pediatrics*, 70, 539–46.

Hingson, R., Howland, J. and Winter, M. (1989). 'Characteristics of persons who ride with drunk drivers: results of a Massachusetts survey of adolescents and adults', Paper presented at Kettil Bruun Society Symposium, Maastricht, Netherlands.

Hingson, R., Strunin, L. and Berlin, B. (1990). 'Changes in knowledge and behaviors among adolescents, Massachusetts Statewide Surveys, 1986–1988', *Pediatrics*, 85, 24–9.

Hingson, R., Strunin, L., Berlin, B. and Heeren, T. (1990). 'Beliefs about AIDS, use of alcohol, drugs and unprotected sex among Massachusetts adolescents', *American Journal of Public Health*, 80, 295–9.

Holgate, H. (1990). *Young People's Perceptions of HIV/AIDS*, North West Surrey Health Authority, Health Promotion Service.

Holmila, M. (1988). *Wives, Husbands and Alcohol*, Helsinki, Finnish Foundation for Alcohol Studies.

Home Office (1987). *Young People and Alcohol: Report of the Working Group*, Standing Conference on Crime Prevention, London, Home Office.

Home Office (1979–90). *Statistics of the Misuse of Drugs*, Bulletins, London, Home Office.

Home Office (1990a). *Offences of Drunkenness, England and Wales 1989*. Statistical Bulletin 40/90, London, Home Office.

Home Office (1990b). *Statistics of the Misuse of Drugs: Addicts Notified to the Home Office, United Kingdom, 1989*, Statistical Bulletin 7/90, London, Home Office.

Home Office (1990c). *Statistics of the Misuse of Drugs: Seizures and Offenders*

Dealt With, United Kingdom, 1989, Statistical Bulletin 24/90, London, Home Office.

Home Office (1991). *Statistics of the Misuse of Drugs: Addicts Notified to the Home Office, United Kingdom, 1990*, Statistical Bulletin 8/91, London, Home Office.

Homel, R. (1988). *Policing and Punishing the Drinking Driver*, New York, Springer-Verlag.

Humphries, S. (1991). *A Secret World of Sex*, London, Sidgwick & Jackson.

Hundleby, J., Carpenter, R., Ross, R. and Mercer, G. (1982). 'Adolescent drug use and other behaviors', *Journal of Child Psychology and Psychiatry*, 23, 61–8.

Hunt, A.J., Davies, P.M., Weatherburn, P., Coxon, A.P.M. and McManus, T.J. (1991). 'Changes in sexual behaviour in a large cohort of homosexual men in England and Wales 1988–9', *British Medical Journal*, 302, 505–6.

Independent Scientific Committee on Smoking and Health (1987). *Interim Statement on Passive Smoking*, London, Hansard 1986/87, 112, cols. 326–7 w (13 March).

Inglis, B. (1975). *The Forbidden Game: A Social History of Drugs*, London, Hodder & Stoughton.

Irwin, C.E. (1989). 'Risk-taking behaviors in the adolescent patient: are they impulsive?', *Pediatric Annals*, 18, 122–33.

Irwin, C.E. and Millstein, S.G. (1986). 'Biopsychosocial correlates of risk-taking behaviors during adolescence', *Journal of Adolescent Health Care*, 7, 825–965.

Ives, R. (ed.) (1986). *Solvent Misuse in Context*, London, National Children's Bureau.

Jabez, A. (1990). 'Crack babies', *Nursing Times*, 18, 18–19.

Jack, M.S. (1989). 'Personal Fable: a potential explanation for risk-taking behavior in adolescents', *Journal of Pediatric Nursing*, 4, 334–8.

Jacobs, M.R. and Fehr, K. O'B. (1987). *Drugs and Drug Abuse: A Reference Text*, Ontario, Addiction Research Foundation.

Jacobson, B. (1988). *Beating the Ladykillers: Women and Smoking*, London, Gollancz.

Jahoda, G. and Cramond, J. (1972). *Children and Alcohol: A Developmental Study in Glasgow*, London, HMSO.

Jahoda, G., Davies, J. and Tagg, S. (1980). 'Parents' alcohol consumption and children's knowledge of drinks and usage patterns', *British Journal of Addiction*, 75, 297–303.

James, N.J., Gillies, P.A. and Bignell, C.J. (1991). 'AIDS-related risk perception and sexual behaviour amongst sexually transmitted disease clinic attenders', *International Journal of STD and AIDS*, 2, 264–71.

Jamieson, A., Glanz, A. and MacGregor, S. (1984). *Dealing With Drug Misuse*, London, Tavistock.

Janz, N.K. and Becker, M.H. (1984). 'The Health Belief Model: a decade later', *Health Education Quarterly*, 11, 1–47.

Jeffrey, C.G. (1970). 'Drug control in the United Kingdom'. In: Phillipson, R.V. (ed.) *Modern Trends in Drug Dependence and Alcoholism*, London, Butterworths, pp. 60–74.

Jenny, C. (1988). 'Adolescent risk-taking behavior and the occurrence of sexual assault', *American Journal of the Diseases of Children*, 142, 770–2.

Jessor, R. (1987). 'Problem-Behaviour Theory, psychological development, and adolescent problem drinking', *British Journal of Addiction*, 82, 331–42.

Jessor, R. (1989). 'Road safety and health behavior: some lessons for research and intervention', *Health Education Research*, 5, 281–3.

Jessor, R. (1991). 'Risk behavior in adolescence: a psychosocial framework for understanding and action', personal communication.

Jessor, R., Chase, J.A. and Donovan, J.E. (1980). 'Psychosocial correlates of marijuana use and problem drinking in a national sample of adolescents', *American Journal of Public Health*, 70, 604–13.

Jessor, R., Donovan, J.E. and Costa, F. (1990). 'Personality, perceived life chances, and adolescent health behavior'. In: Hurrelmann, K. and Losel, F. (eds) *Health Hazards in Adolescence*, New York, Walter de Gruyter, pp. 25–41.

Jessor, R., Donovan, J.E. and Costa, F.M. (1991). *Beyond Adolescence*, Cambridge, Cambridge University Press.

Jessor, R. and Jessor, S.L. (1977). *Problem Behavior and Psychosocial Development: A Longitudinal Study of Youth*, New York, Academic Press.

Jessor, R. and Jessor, S.L. (1984). 'Adolescence to young adulthood: a 12-year perspective study of problem behavior and psychosocial development'. In: Mednick, S.A., Harway, M. and Finello, K.M. (eds) *Handbook of Longitudinal Research*, Vol. 2, *Teenage and Adult Cohorts*, New York, Praeger, pp. 34–61.

Johnson, A.M., Wadsworth, J., Elliott, P., Prior, L., Wallace, P., Blower, S., Webb, N.L., Heald, G.I., Miller, D.L., Adler, M.W. and Anderson, R.M. (1989). 'A pilot study of sexual lifestyles in a random sample of the population of Great Britain', *AIDS*, 3, 135–41.

Johnson, S.F., McCarter, R.J. and Ferencz, C. (1987). 'Changes in alcohol, cigarette and recreational drug use during pregnancy: implications for intervention', *American Journal of Epidemiology*, 126, 695–702.

Jonah, B.A. (1986). 'Accident risks and risk-taking behaviour among young drivers', *Accidents: Annals and Prevention*, 18, 255–71.

Jones, K.L. and Smith, D.W. (1973). 'Recognition of the foetal alcohol syndrome in early infancy', *Lancet*, II, 999–1001.

Jones, K.L., Smith, D.W., Ulleland, C.N. and Streissguth, A.P. (1973). 'Patterns of malformation in offspring of chronic alcoholic mothers', *Lancet*, I, 1267–71.

Judson, H.F. (1973). *Heroin Addiction in Britain*, London, Harcourt Brace Jovanovich.

Kahn, J.R., Kahbech, W.D. and Hofferth, S.L. (1988). 'National estimates of teenage sexual activity: evaluating the comparability of three national surveys', *Demography*, 25, 189–204.

Kalant, O.J. (ed.) (1980). *Alcohol and Drug Problems in Women*, New York, Plenum.

Kalb, M. (1975). 'The myth of alcoholism prevention', *Preventive Medicine*, 4, 404–16.

Kaminski, M., Franc, M., Lebouvier, M., Dumaxanbrun, C. and Rumeau-Roquette, C. (1981). 'Moderate alcohol use and pregnancy outcome', *Neurobehavioural Toxicology and Teratology*, 3, 173–81.

Kandel, D.B. (1978). *Longitudinal Research on Drug Use*, New York, Halstead.

Kandel, D.B. and Logan, J.A. (1984). 'Patterns of drug use from adolescence to young adulthood. I. Periods of risk for initiation, continued use and discontinuation', *American Journal of Public Health*, 74, 660–6.

Kaplan, H.S. (1974). *The New Sex Therapy*, Harmondsworth, Pelican.

Kegeles, S.M., Adler, N.E. and Irwin, C.E. (1988). 'Sexually active adolescents and condoms: changes over one year in knowledge, attitudes and use', *American Journal of Public Health*, 78, 460–1.

Kiianmaa, K., Tabakoff, B. and Saito, T. (eds) (1989). *Genetic Aspects of Alcoholism*, Helsinki, Finnish Foundation for Alcohol Studies.

Kinder, B.N., Pape, N.E. and Walfish, S. (1980). 'Drug and alcohol education programmes: a review of outcome studies', *International Journal of the Addictions*, 15, 1035–54.

Kinsey, A.C., Pomeroy, W.B. and Martin, C.E. (1948). *Sexual Behavior in the Human Male*, Philadelphia, W.B. Saunders.

Kinsey, A.C., Pomeroy, W.B., Martin, C.E. and Gebhard, P.H. (1953). *Sexual Behavior in the Human Female*, Philadelphia, W.B. Saunders.

Klee, H., Faugier, J., Hayes, C., Boulton, T. and Morris, J. (1990). 'Sexual partners of injecting drug users: the risk of HIV infection', *British Journal of Addiction*, 85, 413–18.

Klee, H., Faugier, J., Hayes, C. and Morris, J. (1991). 'Risk reduction among injecting drug users: changes in the sharing of injecting equipment and in condom use', *AIDS Care*, 3, 63–73.

Klepp, K-I. and Perry, C.L. (1990). 'Adolescents, drinking and driving: who doesn't and why?'. In: Wilson, R.J. and Mann, R.E. (eds) *Drinking and Driving*, London, Guilford, pp. 42–67.

Knupfer, G. (1991). 'Abstaining for foetal health: the fiction that even light drinking is dangerous', *British Journal of Addiction*, 86, 1063–74.

Kosviner, A. and Hawks, D (1977). 'Cannabis use amongst British university students, II. Patterns of use and attitudes to use', *British Journal of Addiction*, 72, 41–58.

Kozlowski, L.T. (1991). 'Rehabilitating a genetic perspective in the study of tobacco and alcohol use', *British Journal of Addiction*, 86, 517–20.

Kraft, J. (1970). 'Drug addiction and personality disorder', *British Journal of Addiction*, 64, 403–8.

Kreitman, N. (1986). 'Alcohol consumption and the preventive paradox', *British Journal of Addiction*, 81, 353–64.

Kulstad, R. (ed.) (1988). *AIDS 1988*, Washington, DC, American Association for the Advancement of Science.

Kuzma, J. and Sokol, R. (1982). 'Maternal drinking behaviour and decreased intrauterine growth', *Alcoholism, Clinical and Experimental Research*, 6, 396–402.

Lacey, R. and Woodward, S. (1985). *That's Life Survey on Tranquillisers*, London, BBC.

Lane, D.A. (1976). 'Predictors of drug use', *Community Health*, 8, 12–15.

Leathar, D.S., Hastings, G.B. and Squair, S.I. (1985). *Evaluation of the Scottish Health Education Group's 1985 Drug Abuse Campaign*, Advertising Research Unit, University of Strathclyde.

Leck, P., McEwan, J., Moreton, W. *et al.* (1985). *Action on Smoking at Work*, London, Academic Department of Community Medicine, King's College School of Medicine and Dentistry.

Leigh, B.C. (1990a). '"Venus gets in my thinking": drinking and female sexuality in the age of AIDS', *Journal of Substance Abuse*, 2, 129–45.

Leigh, B.C. (1990b). 'Alcohol use and sexual behavior in discrete events: II. Comparison of three samples', Paper presented at the Alcohol Epidemiology Symposium, Kettil Bruun Society, Budapest, Hungary.

Leigh, B.C. (1990c). 'The relationship of substance use during sex to high-risk sexual behavior', *The Journal of Sex Research*, 27, 199–213.

Leigh, B.C. (1990d). 'The relationship of sex-related alcohol expectancies to alcohol consumption and sexual behavior', *British Journal of Addiction*, 85, 919–28.

Leitenberg, H., Greenwald, E. and Tarran, M.J. (1989). 'The relation between sexual activity among children during preadolescence and/or early adolescence and sexual behavior and sexual adjustment in young adulthood', *Archives of Sexual Behavior*, 18, 299–313.

Lemoine, P., Harronsseau, H., Borteyrou, J.P. and Menure, J.C. (1968). 'Les enfants de parents alcooliques: anomalies observées à propos 127 cas', *Ouest médicale*, 25, 476–82.

Lepage, P., Vande Perre, P., Carael, M., Nsengumudeny, F., Njarunzrza, J., Butzler, J. and Sprecher, S. (1987). 'Postnatal transmission of HIV from mother to child', *Lancet*, II, 400.

Lester, B. (1989). *Women and AIDS*, New York, Continuum.

Lipson, A.H. and Webster, W.S. (1990). 'Response to letters dealing with warning labels on alcoholic beverages', *Teratology*, 41, 479–81.

Little, R.E. (1977). 'Moderate alcohol use during pregnancy and decreased infant birth weight', *American Journal of Public Health*, 67, 1154–6.

Little, R.E., Streissguth, A.P. and Guzinski, G.M. (1981). 'Prevention of fetal alcohol syndrome: a model program', *Alcoholism: Clinical and Experimental Research*, 4, 185–9.

McAlistair, A., Perry, C., Killen, J., Simkard, L.A. and Maudsy, N. (1981). 'Pilot study of smoking, alcohol and drug abuse prevention', *American Journal of Public Health*, 70, 719–25.

MacAndrew, C. and Edgerton, R.B. (1970). *Drunken Comportment: A Social Explanation*, London, Nelson.

MacArthur, C., Newton, J.R. and Knox, E.G. (1987). 'Effect of anti-smoking health education on infant size at birth: a randomized control trial', *British Journal of Obstetrics and Gynaecology*, 94, 295–300.

McConville, B. (1983). *Women under the Influence*, London, Virago.

McDonald, A. (1984). 'The meaning of risk–taking behaviour', *Australian Family Physician*, 13, 42–4.

McEwan, R., McCallum, A., Bhopal, R.S. and Madnok, R. (1991). 'Sex and HIV infection: the role of alcohol', personal communication.

McGarry, J. (1989). 'Sexual behaviour of young women', *British Medical Journal*, 298, 1453.

MacGregor, S. (ed.) (1989). *Drugs and British Society*, London, Routledge.

McKay, A.J., Hawthorne, V.M. and McCartney, H.N. (1973). 'Drug taking amongst medical students at Glasgow University', *British Medical Journal*, 1, 540–3.

McKechnie, R., Cameron, D., Cameron, I. and Drewery, J. (1977). 'Teenage drinking in South-West Scotland', *British Journal of Addiction*, 72, 287–95.

McKeganey, N., Barnard, M. and Watson, H. (1989). 'HIV-related risk behaviour among a non-clinic sample of injecting drug users', *British Journal of Addiction*, 84, 1481–90.

McKennell, A.C. and Thomas, R.K. (1967). *Adults' and Adolescents' Smoking Habits and Attitudes*, London, HMSO.

McKirnan, D.J. and Peterson, P.L. (1989). 'Alcohol and drug use amongst homosexual men and women: epidemiology and population characteristics', *Addictive Behaviors* 14, 545–53.

McKnight, A. and Merrett, D. (1987). 'Alcohol consumption in pregnancy – a health education problem', *Journal of the Royal College of General Practitioners*, 37, 73–6.

MacLennan, A. (ed.) (1976). *Women: Their Use of Alcohol and Other Legal Drugs*, Toronto, Addiction Research Foundation.

McMillan, A. (1989). 'Sexually transmitted diseases', *Pulse*, 7 October, 49–54.

McMillan, A. (1991). Personal communication.

McQueen, D., Robertson, B.J. and Smith, R.J. (1988). *AIDS-Related Behaviours in Scotland: Provisional Data from the RUHBC CATI Survey*, Edinburgh, Research Unit in Health and Behaviour Change (RUHBC Report No. 2).

Majewski, F. (1981). 'Alcohol embryopathology: some facts and speculations about pathogenesis', *Neurobehavioural Toxicology and Teratology*, 3, 129–44.

Malcolm, S. and Shephard, R. (1978). 'Personalized and sexual behavior of the adolescent smoker', *American Journal of Drug and Alcohol Abuse*, 5, 87–96.

Mant, D., Vessey, M. and London, N. (1988). 'Social class differences in sexual behaviour and cervical cancer', *Community Medicine*, 10, 52–6.

Marsh, A., Dobbs, J. and White, A. (1986). *Adolescent Drinking*, London, HMSO.

Marsh, C. (1986). 'Medicine and the media', *British Medical Journal*, 292, 895.

Martin, T.R. and Bracken, M.B. (1986). 'Association of low birth weight with passive smoke exposure in pregnancy', *American Journal of Epidemiology*, 124, 633–42.

Masters, W.H., Johnson, V.E. and Kolodny, R.C. (1988). *Crisis: Heterosexual Behavior in the Age of AIDS*, London, Grafton.

Matza, D. (1964). *Delinquency and Drift*, New York, Wiley.

Matza, D. (1969). *Becoming Deviant*, Englewood Cliffs, NJ, Prentice-Hall.

May, C. (1991). 'Research on alcohol education for young people: review of the literature', *Health Education Journal*, 50, 195–9.

Maynard, A. and Tether, P. (eds) (1990). *Preventing Alcohol and Tobacco Problems*, Vol. 1, Aldershot, Avebury.

Melotte, C. (1975). 'A rehabilitation hostel for drug users: one year's admissions', *British Journal of Criminology*, 15, 376–85.

Mena, M.R., Albornoz, C., Puente, M. and Moreno, C. (1980). 'Sindrome fetal alcoholico', *Revsila Chilena de Pediatria*, 51, 414–23.

Mills, J.L. and Granbard, B.I. (1987). 'Is moderate drinking during pregnancy associated with an increased risk of malformations?', *Pediatrics*, 80, 309–14.

Montague, A. (1965). *Life Before Birth*, New York, Signet, p. 114.

Morgan Thomas, R. (1990). 'AIDS risks, alcohol, drugs and the sex industry: a Scottish study'. In: Plant, M.A. (ed.) *AIDS, Drugs and Prostitution*, London, Tavistock/Routledge, pp. 88–108.

Morgan Thomas, R., Plant, M.A. and Plant, M.L. (1990). 'Alcohol, AIDS risks and sex industry clients: results from a Scottish study', *Drug and Alcohol Dependence*, 26, 265–9.

Morgan Thomas, R., Plant, M.A., Plant, M.L. and Sales, J. (1990). 'Risk of HIV infection among clients of the sex industry in Scotland', *British Medical Journal*, 301, 525.

MORI (1990). *Teenage Smoking*, London, MORI.

Morrison, V. (1991). 'The impact of HIV upon injecting drug users: a longitudinal study', *AIDS Care*, 3, 197–205.

Morrison, V. and Plant, M.A. (1990). 'Drug problems and patterns of service use amongst illicit drug users in Edinburgh', *British Journal of Addiction*, 85, 547–54.

Morrison, V. and Plant, M.A. (1991). 'Licit and illicit drug initiations and alcohol-related problems amongst illicit drug users in Edinburgh', *Drug and Alcohol Dependence*, 27, 19–27.

Mort, F. (1987). *Dangerous Sexualities*, London, Routledge & Kegan Paul.

Mott, F.L. and Haurin, R.J. (1988). 'Linkages between sexual activity and alcohol and drug use among American adolescents', *Family Planning Perspectives*, 20, 128–36.

Mott, J. (1976). 'The epidemiology of self-reported drug misuse in the United Kingdom', *Bulletin on Narcotics*, 28, 43–54.

Mott, J. (1989). 'Self-reported cannabis use in Great Britain in 1981', *British Journal of Addiction*, 80, 30–43.

Murray, M., Swan, A.V., Bewley, B.R. and Johnson, M.R.D. (1983). 'The development of smoking during adolescence', *International Journal of Epidemiology*, 12, 185–92.

Myers, T. (1982). *Alcohol and Crimes of Interpersonal Violence*, PhD thesis, University of Edinburgh.

Myers, T. (1983). 'Alcohol and violence: self-reported alcohol consumption amongst violent and non-violent male prisoners', *British Journal of Addiction*, 77, 399–413.

Myers, T. (1986). 'An analysis of context and alcohol consumption in a group of criminal events', *Alcohol and Alcoholism*, 21, 389–95.

National Research Council (1986). *Environmental Tobacco Smoke*, Washington, National Academy Press.

National Research Council (1989). *AIDS: Sexual Behavior and Intravenous Drug Use*. Washington, National Academy Press.

Neubauer, B.J. (1989). 'Risk-taking, responsibility for health and attitude toward avoiding AIDS', *Psychological Reports*, 64, 1255–60.

Niewoehner, D.E., Kleinerman, J. and Rice, D.B. (1974). 'Pathogenic changes in the peripheral airways of young smokers', *New England Journal of Medicine*, 291, 755–8.

NOP Market Research Ltd. (1982). 'Survey of drug use in the 15–21 age group undertaken by the *Daily Mail*', London, NOP.

O'Connor, J. (1978). *The Young Drinkers*, London, Tavistock.

Office of Population Censuses and Surveys (1980). *General Household Survey 1978*, London, HMSO.

Office of Population Censuses and Surveys (1990). *Mortality Statistics, England and Wales 1988*, London, HMSO.

Ogborne, A.C. (1975). 'The first 100 residents in a therapeutic community for former addicts', *British Journal of Addiction*, 70, 65–76.

Okun, M., Stock, W.A. and Ceurvorst, R.W. (1980). 'Risk taking through the adult life span', *Experimental Ageing Research*, 6, 463–73.

Olegard, R., Sabel, K.G., Aronsson, M., Sandia, B., Johansson, P.R., Carlsson, C., Kyllerman, M., Inverssa, K. and Horbeck, A. (1979). 'Effects on the child of alcohol abuse during pregnancy', *Acta Paediatrica Scandinavica Supplementum* 275, 112–21.

Olenckno, W.A. and Blacconiere, M.J. (1990). 'Risk-taking behaviors and other correlates of seat belt use among university students', *Public Health*, 104, 155–64.

Olsen, J. (1991). 'Does maternal tobacco smoking modify the effect of alcohol on fetal growth?', *American Journal of Public Health*, 81, 69–73.

O'Reilly, K.R. and Aral, S.O. (1985). 'Adolescent sexual behavior', *Journal of Adolescent Health Care*, 6, 262–70.

Orford, J. (1985). *Excessive Appetites: A Psychological View of Addictions*, Chichester, Wiley.

Orford, J. and Harwin, J. (eds) (1982). *Alcohol and the Family*, London, Croom Helm.

Pahava, R., Good, R. and Pahava, S. (1987). 'Prematurity, hypogammaglobulinemia and neuropathology with human immunodeficiency virus (HIV) infection', *Proceedings of the National Academy of Sciences*, 84, 3826–30.

Parker, D.A., Harford, T.C. and Rosenstock, G.M. (1990). 'Alcohol, other drugs and sexual risk-taking among young adults in the United States', Paper presented at the Alcohol Epidemiology Symposium, Kettil Bruun Society, Budapest, Hungary.

Parker, H., Bakx, K. and Newcombe, R. (1988). *Living with Heroin*, Milton Keynes, Open University Press.

Partanen, J. (1991). *Sociability and Intoxication*, Helsinki, Finnish Foundation for Alcohol Studies.

Partanen, J., Bruun, K. and Markkanen, T. (1966). *Inheritance of Drinking Behaviour*, Helsinki, Finnish Foundation for Alcohol Studies.

Pattison, C.J., Barnes, E.A. and Thorley, A. (1982). *South Tyneside Drug Prevalence and Indicator Study*, Newcastle, Centre for Drug and Alcohol Studies.

Peacock, C. (1992). 'International policies on drinking and driving: a review', *International Journal of the Addictions*, 27, 187–208.

Pearson, G. (1987). *The New Heroin Users*, Oxford, Blackwell.

Pearson, G., Gilman, M. and MacIver, S. (1985). *Young People and Heroin Use in the North of England*, London, Health Education Council Report.

Peck, D.F. (1982). 'Problem drinking: some determining factors'. In: Plant, M.A. (ed.) *Drinking and Problem Drinking*, London, Junction, pp. 65–83.

Peckham, C.S. and Newell, M-L (1990). 'HIV-1 infection in mothers and babies', *AIDS Care*, 2, 205–11.

Pederson, W. (1990). 'Drinking games adolescents play', *British Journal of Addiction*, 85, 1483–90.

Peluso, E. and Peluso, L.S. (1988). *Women and Drugs*, Annapolis, Comp Care Publishers.

Pickens, K. (1983). 'Drug education: the effects of giving information', *Journal of Drug Education*, 13, 32–44.

Pittman, D.J. and Snyder, C.R. (eds) (1962). *Society, Culture and Drinking Patterns*, New York, Wiley.

Plant, M.A. (1973). *Young People at Risk: A Study of the 17–24 Age Group*, Cheltenham, Cheltenham Youth Trust (unpublished report).

Plant, M.A. (1975). *Drugtakers in an English Town*, London, Tavistock.

Plant, M.A. (1981). 'What aetiologies?'. In: Edwards, G. and Busch, C. (eds) *Drug Problems in Britain*, London, Academic Press, pp. 249–80.

Plant, M.A. (1987). *Drugs in Perspective*, London, Hodder & Stoughton.

Plant, M.A. (ed.) (1990). *AIDS, Drugs and Prostitution*, London, Tavistock/ Routledge.

Plant, M.A., Bagnall, G. and Foster, J. (1990). 'Teenage heavy drinkers: alcohol-related knowledge, beliefs, experiences, motivation and the social context of drinking', *Alcohol and Alcoholism*, 25, 691–8.

Plant, M.A., Bagnall, G., Foster, J. and Sales, J. (1990a). 'Young people and drinking: results of an English national survey', *Alcohol and Alcoholism*, 25, 685–90.

Plant, M.A. and Foster, J. (1991). 'Teenagers and alcohol: results of a Scottish national survey', *Drug and Alcohol Dependence*, 28, 203–10.

Plant, M.A., Goos, C., Keup, W. and Osterberg, E. (eds) (1990b). *Alcohol and Drugs: Research and Policy*, Edinburgh, Edinburgh University Press.

Plant, M.A., Grant, M. and Williams, R. (eds.) (1981). *Economics and Alcohol*, London, Croom Helm.

Plant, M.A., Peck, D.F. and Samuel, E. (1985). *Alcohol, Drugs and School-leavers*, London, Tavistock.

Plant, M.A. and Pirie, F. (1979). 'Self-reported alcohol consumption and alcohol-related problems: a study in four Scottish towns', *Social Psychiatry*, 14, 65–73.

Plant, M.A., Ritson, E.B. and Robertson, J.R. (eds) (1992). *Alcohol and Drugs: The Scottish Experience*, Edinburgh, Edinburgh University Press.

Plant, M.L. (1985). *Women, Drinking and Pregnancy*, London, Tavistock.

Plant, M.L. (1988). 'Drinking and pregnancy: a review', *International Clinical Nutrition Review*, 8, 12–17.

Plant, M.L. (1990). 'Maternal alcohol and tobacco use during pregnancy'. In: Alexander, J., Levy, V. and Roch, S. (eds) *Antenatal Care: A Research-Based Approach*, London, Macmillan, pp. 73–87.

Plant, M.L. (1990). *Women and Alcohol*, Copenhagen, World Health Organization Regional Office for Europe.

Plant, M.L. (1991). 'Alcohol and breast cancer: a review', *International Journal of the Addictions*, 27, 107–28.

Plant, M.L., Plant, M.A. and Morgan Thomas, R. (1990). 'Alcohol, AIDS risks and commercial sex: some preliminary results from a Scottish study', *Drug and Alcohol Dependence*, 25, 51–5.

Porter, R., O'Connor, M. and Whelan, J. (eds) (1984). *Mechanisms of Alcohol Damage in Utero*, London, Pitman.

Poskitt, E.M.E., Hensey, O.J. and Smith, C.S. (1982). 'Alcohol, other drugs and the foetus', *Developmental Medicine and Child Neurology*, 24, 596–602.

Pritchard, C., Fielding, M., Choudry, N., Cox, M. and Diamond, I. (1986). 'Incidence of drug and solvent abuse in "normal" fourth and fifth year comprehensive school children – some socio-behavioural characteristics', *British Journal of Social Work*, 16, 341–51.

Raistrick, D. and Davidson, R. (1985). *Alcoholism and Drug Addiction*, Edinburgh, Churchill Livingstone.

Ray, B.A. and Brande, M.D. (1986). *Women and Drugs: A New Era for Research*, Rockville, Maryland, National Institute on Drug Abuse.

Registrar General Scotland (1988). *Annual Report 1987*, Edinburgh, HMSO.

Registrar General Scotland (1989). *Annual Report 1988*, Edinburgh, HMSO.

Remafedi, G.J. (1988). 'Preventing the sexual transmission of AIDS during adolescence', *Journal of Adolescent Health Care*, 9, 139–43.

Revkin, A.C. (1989). 'Crack in the cradle', *Discover*, September, 62–9.

Ridlon, F.V.C. (1988). *A Fallen Angel: The Status Insularity of the Female Alcoholic*, London, Bricknell University Press.

Ritson, E.B. (1981). 'Alcohol and young people', *Journal of Adolescence*, 4, 93–100.

Robertson, J.A. (1990). *The Role of Alcohol and Illicit Drugs in the Marital Adjustment of Young People*, MPhil thesis, University of Edinburgh.

Robertson, J.A. and Plant, M.A. (1988). 'Alcohol, sex and risk of HIV infection', *Drug and Alcohol Dependence*, 22, 75–8.

Robertson, J.R. (1987). *Heroin, AIDS and Society*, London, Hodder & Stoughton.

Robinson, D., Maynard, A. and Chester, R. (eds) (1989). *Controlling Legal Addictions*, London, Macmillan.

Rona, R.J., Chin, S. and Du V Florey, C. (1985). 'Exposure to cigarette smoking and children's growth', *International Journal of Epidemiology*, 14, 402–9.

Room, R. (1983). 'Introduction'. In: Room, R. and Collins, G. (eds) *Alcohol and Disinhibition: Nature and Meaning of the Link*, Washington DC, NIAAA, Research Monograph 12, US Department of Health and Human Services.

Roquette, P.C. (1957). *The Influence of Parental Alcohol Toxicomania on the Physical and Mental Development of Young Children*, MD Thesis, University of Paris.

Roscoe, B., Cavanaugh, L.E. and Kennedy, D.R. (1988). 'Dating infidelity: behaviors, reasons and consequences', *Adolescence*, 23, 35–43.

Rose, G. (1981). 'Strategy of prevention: lessons from cardiovascular diseases', *British Medical Journal*, 282, 1847–91.

Rosenbaum, M. (1981). *Women on Heroin*, New Brunswick, NJ, Rutgers University Press.

Rosenberg, M. (ed.) (1987). *Smoking and Reproductive Health*, Massachusetts, PSG.

Rosett, H.L. (1977). 'The pre-natal clinic: a site for alcoholism prevention and treatment'. In: Seixas, F.A. (ed.) *Currents in Alcoholism*, New York, Grune & Stratton, p. 419.

Rosett, H.L., Ouellette, E.M., Weiner, L. and Owens, E. (1978). 'Therapy of heavy drinking during pregnancy', *American Journal of Obstetrics and Gynaecology*, 51, 41.

Rosett, H.L. and Weiner, L. (1984). *Alcohol and the Fetus*, New York, Oxford University Press.

Rosett, H.L., Weiner, L. and Edelin, K.C. (1983). 'Treatment experience with pregnant problem drinkers', *Journal of the American Medical Association*, 249, 2029–33.

Rosett, H.L., Weiner, L., Lee, A., Zuckerman, B., Dooling, E. and Oppenheimer, E. (1983). 'Patterns of alcohol consumption and fetal development', *Obstetrics and Gynaecology*, 61, 539–46.

Rosett, H.L., Weiner, L., Zuckerman, B., McKinlay, S. and Edelin, K.C. (1980). 'Reduction of alcohol consumption during pregnancy with benefits to the newborn', *Alcoholism: Clinical and Experimental Research*, 4, 178–84.

Ross, H.L. (1982). *Deterring the Drinking Driver*, Lexington, D.C. Heath.

Rotkin, I.D. (1981). 'Etiology and epidemiology of cervical cancer'. In: Dallenbach-Hellwegg, H. (ed.) *Current Topics in Pathology – Cervical Cancer*, Berlin, Springer-Verlag, pp. 81–110.

Royal College of General Practitioners (1986). *Alcohol: A Balanced View*, London, Royal College of General Practitioners.

Royal College of Obstetricians and Gynaecologists (1991). *Report of the Working Party on Unplanned Pregnancy*, London, Chamelion Press.

Royal College of Physicians (1977). *Smoking or Health*, London, Pitman.

Royal College of Physicians (1986). *Health or Smoking?*, London, Pitman.

Royal College of Physicians (1987). *A Great and Growing Evil: The Medical Consequences of Alcohol Abuse*, London, Tavistock.

Royal College of Psychiatrists (1986). *Alcohol: Our Favourite Drug*, London, Tavistock.

Royal College of Psychiatrists (1987). *Drug Scenes*, London, Gaskell.

Rubin, D.H., Krasilnikoff, P.A., Leventhal, J.M., Weil, B. and Berget, A. (1986). 'Effect of passive smoking on birth weight', *Lancet*, II, 415–17.

Rubin, P.C. (1986). 'The use of drugs, alcohol and cigarettes during pregnancy', *British Medical Journal*, 292, 696.

Rubin, P.C. (ed.) (1987). *Prescribing in Pregnancy*, London, British Medical Journal.

Rubin, P.C., Craig, G.F., Gavin, K. and Sumner, D. (1986). 'Prospective survey of use of therapeutic drugs, alcohol and cigarettes during pregnancy', *British Medical Journal*, 292, 81–3.

Russell, M. (1974). 'The smoking habit and its classification', *The Practitioner*, 212, 791–800.

Sales, J., Duffy, J., Plant, M.A. and Peck, D.F. (1989). 'Alcohol consumption, cigarette sales and mortality in the United Kingdom: an analysis of the period 1970–1985', *Drug and Alcohol Dependence*, 24, 155–60.

Saucier, J-F. and Ambert, A-M. (1983). 'Parental marital status and adolescents' health-risk behavior', *Adolescence*, 18, 403–11.

Schaps, E., Dibartolo, R., Moskowitz, J., Balley, C.G. and Churgin, G. (1981). 'A review of 127 drug abuse prevention programme evaluations', *Journal of Drug Issues*, 11, 17–43.

Schilts, R. (1987). *And the Band Played On*, Harmondsworth, Penguin.

Scheifer, S., Keller, S.E., Franklin, J.E., Lafarce, S. and Miller, S. (1990). 'HIV zeropositivity in inner-city alcoholics', *Hospital and Community Psychiatry*, 41, 248–54.

Schofield, M. (1973). *The Sexual Behaviour of Young Adults*, London, Allen Lane.

Schuckit, M.A. (ed.) (1985). *Alcohol Patterns and Problems*, New Brunswick, NJ, Rutgers University Press.

Seegmiller, R.E., Carey, J.C. and Fineman, R.M. (1987). 'The hazards of drinking alcoholic beverages during pregnancy: should the public be warned?', *Teratology*, 35, 479.

Seely, J.E., Zuskin, E. and Bonhuys, A. (1971). 'Cigarette smoking: objective evidence for lung damage in teenagers', *Science*, 172, 741–3.

Segal, B. (1988). *Drugs and Behavior*, New York, Gardner Press.

Seltzer, V.L., Rabin, J. and Benjamin, F. (1989). 'Teenagers' awareness of the Acquired Immunodeficiency Syndrome and the impact on their sexual behavior', *Obstetrics and Gynaecology*, 74, 55–8.

Sexton, M. and Habel, J.R. (1984). 'A clinical trial of change in maternal smoking and its effect on birth weight', *Journal of the American Medical Association*, 251, 911–15.

Shapiro, H. (1989). 'Crack – the story so far', *Health Education Journal*, 48, 140–4.

Shapiro, H. (1989). *Drugs in Sport*, London, Gloucester Press.

Sharp, D. and Lowe, G. (1989). 'Adolescents and alcohol – a review of the recent British research', *Journal of Adolescence*, 12, 295–307.

Sherr, L. (1990). 'Pregnancy and paediatrics', *AIDS Care*, 2, 403–8.

Siegel, K., Mesagho, F., Chen, J-Y. and Christ, G. (1989). 'Factors distinguishing homosexual males practising risky and safer sex', *Science and Medicine*, 28, 561–9.

Siegel, L. (ed.) (1987). *AIDS and Substance Abuse*, New York, Harrington Park Press.

Silver, A.M. (1977). 'Some personality characteristics of groups of young drug misusers and delinquents', *British Journal of Addiction*, 72, 143–50.

Simpson, H.M., Mayhew, D.R. and Warren, R.A. (1982). 'Epidemiology of road accidents involving young adults: alcohol, drugs and other factors', *Drug and Alcohol Dependence*, 10, 35–63.

Simpson, J. (1988). *Touching the Void*, London, Jonathan Cape.

Smart, R.G. (1983). *Forbidden Highs*, Toronto, Addiction Research Foundation.

Smith, D.F., Macleod, P.M., Tredwell, G., Wood, B. and Newman, D.E. (1981). 'Intrinsic defects in the fetal alcohol syndrome: studies on 76 cases from British Columbia and the Yukon Territory', *Neurobehavioral Toxicology and Teratology*, 3, 145–52.

Smith, F.O., Arcuri, A.F. and Lester, D. (1987). 'Attitudes toward risk-taking in disadvantaged and academically excellent students', *Perceptual and Motor Skills*, 64, 26.

Smith, R. (1987). *Unemployment and Health*, Oxford, Oxford University Press.

Soloman, D. and Andrews, G. (1973). *Drugs and Sexuality*, Herts, Panther.

Sonenstein, F.L., Pleck, J.H. and Ku, L.C. (1989). 'Sexual activity, condom use and AIDS awareness among adolescent males', *Family Planning Perspectives,* 21, 152–8.

Stall, R. (1988). 'The prevention of HIV infection associated with drug and alcohol use during sexual activity'. In: Siegel, L. (ed.) *AIDS and Substance Abuse*, New York, Harrington Park Press, pp. 73–88.

Stall, R., McKusick, L., Wiley, J. *et al.* (1986). 'Alcohol and drug use during sexual activity and compliance with safe sex guidelines for AIDS: the AIDS Behavioral Research Project', *Health Education Quarterly*, 13, 359–71.

Stall R. and Ostrow, D.A. (1989). 'Intravenous drug use, the combination of drugs and sexual activity and HIV infection among gay and bisexual men: the San Francisco Men's Health Study', *Journal of Drug Issues*, 19, 57–73.

Stangelend, P. (ed.) (1987). *Drugs and Drug Control*, Oxford, Norwegian University Press.

Stimmel, B. (ed.) (1982). *The Effects of Maternal Alcohol and Drug Abuse on the Newborn*, New York, Haworth.

Stimson, G.V. (1981). 'Epidemiological research on drug use in general populations'. In: Edwards, G. and Busch, C. (eds) *Drug Problems in Britain*, London, Academic Press, pp. 51–76.

Stimson, G.V. (1992). 'Drug injecting and HIV infection: new directions for social science research', *International Journal of the Addictions*, 27, 147–64.

Stimson, G.V. and Oppenheimer, E. (1982). *Heroin Addiction*, London, Tavistock.

Stoppard, M. (1982). *Talking Sex*, London, Piccolo.

Strang, J. and Stimson, G.V. (eds) (1990). *AIDS and Drug Misuse*, London, Tavistock/Routledge.

Streissguth, A.P. (1976). 'Psychologic handicaps in children with fetal alcohol syndrome: work in progress on alcoholism', *New York Academy of Science*, 273, 140–5.

Streissguth, A.P., Clarren, S.K. and Jones, K.L. (1985). 'Natural history of the fetal alcohol syndrome', *Lancet*, II, 85–92.

Streissguth, A.P. and Martin, J.C. (1983). 'Prenatal effects of alcohol abuse in human and laboratory animals', *The Pathogenesis of Alcoholism*, 7, New York, Plenum.

Streissguth, A.P., Martin, D.C., Martin, J.C. and Barr, H.M. (1987). 'The Seattle longitudinal prospective study on alcohol and pregnancy', *Neurobehavioral Toxicology and Teratology*, 3, 223–33.

Streissguth, A.P., Sampson, B.D., Barr, H.M., Clarren, S.K. and Martin, D.C.

(1986). 'Studying alcohol teratogenesis from the perspective of the fetal alcohol syndrome: methodological and statistical issues', *Annals of the New York Academy of Sciences*, 477, 63–86.

Strunin, L. and Hingson, R. (1992). 'Alcohol, drugs and adolescent sexual behaviour'. *International Journal of the Addictions*, 27, 129–46.

Suliaman, N., Du V Florey, C. and Taylor, D. (1986). 'The use of drugs, alcohol and cigarettes during pregnancy', *British Medical Journal*, 292, 696.

Sullivan, W.C. (1899). 'A note on the influence of maternal inebriety on the offspring', *Journal of Mental Science*, 45, 489–505.

Sussnam, S., Holt, L., Dent, C.W., Flay, B.R., Graham, J.W., Hansen, W.B. and Johnson, C.A. (1989). 'Activity involvement, risk-taking, demographic variables, and other drug use: prediction of trying smokeless tobacco', *National Cancer Institute Monographs*, 8, 57–62.

Swadi, H. (1988). 'Drug and substance use among 3,333 London adolescents', *British Journal of Addiction*, 83, 935–42.

Swadi, H. (1989). 'Adolescent substance use and truancy: exploring the link', *European Journal of Psychiatry*, 3, 108–15.

Swadi, H. and Zeitlin, H. (1988). 'Peer influence and adolescent substance abuse: a promising side?', *British Journal of Addiction*, 83, 153–8.

Swisher, J.D. (1971). 'Drug education: pushing or preventing?', *Peabody Journal of Education*, 68–79.

Taylor, P. (1984). *Smoke Ring: The Politics of Tobacco*, London, Bodley Head.

Temple, M.T. (1991). 'The relationship between substance use and unsafe sex: a comparison of findings from two samples', Paper presented at the Alcohol Epidemiology Symposium, Kettil Bruun Society, Sigtuna, Sweden.

Temple, M.T. and Leigh, B. (1990). 'Alcohol and sexual behavior in discrete events. I. Characteristics of sexual encounters involving and not involving alcohol', Paper presented at the Alcohol Epidemiology Symposium, Kettil Bruun Society, Budapest, Hungary.

Tether, P. and Robinson, D. (1986). *Preventing Alcohol Problems*, London, Tavistock.

Thomson, E.L. (1978). 'Smoking education programmes 1960–1976', *American Journal of Public Health*, 68, 250–1.

Thorley, A. (1981). 'Longitudinal studies of drug dependence'. In: Edwards, G. and Busch, C. (eds) *Drug Problems in Britain*, London, Academic Press, pp. 117–70.

Thurman, C. (1991). Personal communication.

Tones, K. (1987). 'Role of the health action model in preventing drug abuse', *Health Education Research – Theory and Practice*, 2, 305–16.

Townsend, P. and Davidson, N. (eds) (1988). *Inequalities in Health*, London, Pelican.

Trotter, T. (1813). *An Essay, Medical Philosophical and Chemical on Drunkenness and its Effects on the Human Body*, Boston, Mass., Bradford and Read; republished 1981, New York, Arno Press.

Tuck, M. (1989). *Drinking and Disorder: A Study of Non-Metropolitan Violence*, London, Home Office Research Study 108, HMSO.

Tyler, A. (1986). *Street Drugs*, London, New English Library.

UK Family Planning Research Network (1988). 'Patterns of sexual behaviour amongst sexually experienced women attending family planning clinics in England, Scotland and Wales', *British Journal of Family Planning*, 14, 74–82.

Ulleland, C. (1972). 'The offspring of alcoholic mothers', *Annals of the New York Academy of Sciences*, 197, 167–9.

Ulleland, C., Wennberg, R.P., Igo, R.P. and Smith, N.J. (1970). 'The offspring of alcoholic mothers', *Pediatric Resident*, 4, 474.

United States Surgeon General (1981). 'Advising on alcohol and pregnancy', *Food and Drug Administration Bulletin*, 1, 9–40.

United States Surgeon General (1987). *Children with HIV Infection and Their Families*, Washington, DC, US Department of Health and Human Services.

United States Surgeon General (1988). *Health Consequences of Smoking: Nicotine Addiction*, Washington, DC, Department of Health and Human Services.

Vaillant, G.L. (1983). 'Adolescents, parents, peers: what is one with or without the other?', *Journal of Adolescence*, 6, 131–44.

Wagner, N.W. (ed.) (1974). *Perspectives on Human Sexuality*, New York, Behavioral Publications.

Wald, N., Doll, R. and Copeland, G. (1981). 'Trends in tar, nicotine and carbon monoxide levels of UK cigarettes manufactured since 1934', *British Medical Journal*, 282, 763–5.

Wald, N. and Frogatt, P. (eds) (1988). *Nicotine, Smoking and the Low Tar Programme*, Oxford, Oxford University Press.

Wald, N., Kingluk, S., Darby, S., Doll, R., Pike, M. and Peto, R. (1988). *UK Smoking Statistics*, Oxford, Oxford University Press.

Warburton, D.M. (ed.) (1991). *Addiction Controversies*. Reading, Harwood.

Warner, R.H. and Rosett, H.L. (1975). 'The effects of drinking on offspring', *Journal of Studies on Alcohol*, 36, 1395–420.

Watson, J. (1979). 'Solvent abuse: a retrospective study', *Community Medicine*, 1, 153–6.

Watson, J. (1986). *Solvent Abuse: The Adolescent Epidemic?*, London, Croom Helm.

Weatherburn, P., Davies, P.M., Hunt, A.J., Coxon, A.P.M. and McManus, T.J. (1990). 'Heterosexual behaviour in a large cohort of homosexually active men in England and Wales', *AIDS Care*, 2, 319–24.

Weatherburn, P., Hunt, A.J., Davies, P.M., Coxon, A.P.M. and McManus, T.J. (1991). 'Condom use in a larger cohort of homosexually active men in England and Wales', *AIDS Care*, 3, 31–41.

Weber, T.F., Elfenbein, D.S., Richards, N.L., Davis, A.B. and Thomas, J. (1989). 'Early sexual activity of delinquent adolescents', *Journal of Adolescent Health Care*, 10, 398–403.

Weiner, L., Rosett, H.L., Edelin, K.C., Alpert, J.J. and Zuckerman, B. (1983). 'Alcohol consumption by pregnant women', *Obstetrics and Gynaecology*, 61, 6–12.

Went, D. (1985). *Sex Education for Teachers*, London, Bell & Hyman.

West, R. and Grunberg, N.E. (1991). 'Implications of tobacco use as an addiction', *British Journal of Addiction*, 86, 485–8.

Whittle, M.J. and Hanratty, K.P. (1987). 'Identifying abnormalities'. In: Rubin, P.C. (ed.) *Prescribing in Pregnancy*, London, British Medical Association, pp. 8–18.

Wielardt, H. and Hansen, V.M. (1989). 'Sexual behavior, contraception and unintended pregnancy among young females', *Acta Obstetrica Gynecologica Scandinavica*, 68, 255–9.

Williams, M. (1986). 'The Thatcher generation', *New Society*, 21 February, 312–15.

Wills, J.L. and Branbard, B.I. (1987). 'Is moderate drinking during pregnancy associated with an increased risk of malformations?', *Pediatrics*, 80, 309–14.

Wilson, P. (1980a). 'Drinking habits in the United Kingdom', *Population Trends,* Winter 1980, London, HMSO, pp. 14–18.

Wilson, P. (1980b). *Drinking in England and Wales,* London, HMSO.

Wilson, R.J. and Mann, R.E. (eds) (1990). *Drinking and Driving,* London, Guilford Press.

Windle, M. (1989). 'High risk behaviors for AIDS amongst heterosexual alcoholics', *Journal of Studies on Alcohol,* 50, 503–7.

Wolff, S. (1970). *Children under Stress,* London, Allen Lane.

Woods, S.C. and Mansfield, J.G. (1983). 'Ethanol and disinhibition: physiological and behavioural links'. In: Room, R. and Collins, G. (eds) *Alcohol and Disinhibition: Nature and Meaning of the Link,* Washington, DC, NIAA Research Monograph 12, US Department of Health and Human services, pp. 4–23.

Woodside, M. (1973). 'The first 100 referrals to a Scottish drug addiction treatment centre', *British Journal of Addiction,* 68, 231–41.

World Health Organization (1960). *Epidemiology of Cancer of the Lung,* Geneva, World Health Organization.

World Health Organization (1986). *Tobacco Smoking,* Lyons, International Agency for Research on Cancer.

World Health Organization (1988). *Training on AIDS for Personnel in Drug Treatment Centres,* Copenhagen, World Health Organization.

World Health Organization (1990). *Alcohol Policies: Perspectives from the USSR and Some Other Countries,* Copenhagen, World Health Organization.

World Health Organization (1991). *AIDS among Drug Abusers in Europe,* Copenhagen, World Health Organization.

Wynder, F.L. and Hoffman, D. (1967). *Tobacco and Tobacco Smoke,* New York, Academic Press.

Young, J. (1971). *The Drugtakers,* London, Paladin.

Young, T. (1990). 'Sensation seeking and self-reported criminality among student-athletes', *Perceptual and Motor Skills,* 70, 959–62.

Zelnik, M., Kantner, J.F. and Ford, K. (1981). *Sex and Pregnancy in Adolescence,* Beverly Hills, CA, Sage.

Zuckerman, B. and Hingson, R. (1986). 'Alcohol consumption during pregnancy: a critical review', *Developmental Medicine and Child Neurology,* 28, 649–61.

Name index

Subject index